AI HEALTHCARE WAR ROOM

100 Tactical Approaches to Combat Healthcare Bias and Deploy AI as Your Strategic Health Advisor

Quanda Francis, MBA

Womb WatchAI Corp.

Published by Womb WatchAI Corp. www.wombwatchai.com

First Edition: 2026

ISBN: 979-8-234-06106-5
Ebook 979-8-234-06107-2

Bonus: 100 Ready-to-Use AI Prompts PDF

A Note on the Journal Exercises

This book is designed to be more than something you read — it's designed to be something you DO. At the end of every chapter, you will find two journal exercises that turn the tactical content you just learned into real-world action. Each exercise has a clear prompt, lined writing space for your responses, and a reflection question designed to challenge your thinking.

Do not skip them. The women who get the most out of this book are the ones who complete the exercises honestly — even when the answers are uncomfortable. Especially when the answers are uncomfortable.

If you are reading the **print version**, write directly on the page. This book is meant to be marked up, dog-eared, highlighted, and returned to.

If you are reading on **Kindle Scribe**, you can write your responses directly on the page with the Premium Pen — bringing pen-on-paper feel to your reflection flow on the 11" paper-like display. Use the built-in AI to search, summarize, and uncover insights across your notebook entries as your war room intelligence builds chapter by chapter.

If you are reading on a **phone, tablet, or standard Kindle**, use a notebook or the Notes app on your phone to capture your responses.

Either way, your war room is only as powerful as the intelligence you put into it. Download Rhythm by WOMB WATCHAI® at www.rhythmbywombwatchai.com — your AI health advisor that decodes your lab results, tracks your cycle, analyzes your symptoms, and turns every signal your body sends into the answers you've been waiting your entire life to hear.

Contents

Foreword

In loving memory of my grandmother, Janie

This book is dedicated to my grandmother Janie, whose strength in the face of medical uncertainty shaped my understanding of what it means to advocate for your own health. Throughout her thirties, Grandmother Janie endured heavy bleeding and the debilitating effects of fibroids—symptoms that disrupted her daily life and limited her possibilities in ways that no woman should have to accept.

After years of suffering, she made the difficult decision to undergo a hysterectomy, a choice that finally gave her relief but came only after extensive personal struggle with a healthcare system that offered limited options and little explanation for her family's pattern of reproductive health challenges.

It wasn't until my own traumatic experience during childbirth—when I nearly lost my life—and my subsequent journey through heavy bleeding, multiple gynecologist visits, and endless testing that I began to understand the profound importance of family health history. The key to my diagnosis, and ultimately to better health outcomes, lay not just in my symptoms but in understanding the unique risk factors that ran through generations of women in my family.

This book is written for every woman who has suffered in silence, whose symptoms were dismissed or minimized, who was told that severe pain and disruption were "normal parts of being a woman." It is for those who were misdiagnosed, who lost precious time to medical uncertainty, and tragically, for those we have lost to missed diagnoses of cervical cancer, endometrial cancer, and other conditions that might have been caught earlier with better advocacy and systematic health intelligence.

Most importantly, this book is for every person who refuses to accept that healthcare should be something that happens to them rather than with them. It is for those who understand that their own symptoms, their family patterns, and their research can become powerful tools for achieving better health outcomes.

Grandmother Janie's legacy lives on in the belief that every woman deserves healthcare that listens, understands, and responds to her individual needs. This book carries forward her strength and transforms her struggle into tools that can help others avoid the suffering she endured.

Introduction

FROM PATIENT TO STRATEGIC HEALTH ADVOCATE

The healthcare system was never designed with you in mind. If you're a woman, a person of color, someone with complex symptoms, or anyone who doesn't fit the narrow profile that dominates medical research, you've likely experienced the frustration of medical dismissal, delayed diagnoses, or inadequate care that fails to address your actual health needs.

But here's what the healthcare establishment doesn't want you to know: you can level the playing field using artificial intelligence as your strategic health advisor. This book will teach you to build your AI Healthcare Command Center—a comprehensive system that transforms you from a passive patient into an informed health advocate capable of navigating medical bias, interpreting your symptoms, and communicating effectively with healthcare providers.

The statistics paint a sobering picture. Women are 50% more likely to receive incorrect diagnoses for heart attacks. Black women are three to four times more likely to die from pregnancy-related complications. Patients with rare diseases wait an average of 7.6 years for accurate diagnosis. These aren't isolated incidents—they represent systematic failures in how healthcare approaches anyone who doesn't fit established patterns.

Traditional approaches to healthcare advocacy focus on finding "good doctors" and being "nice patients," hoping that compliance and politeness will lead to better care. This approach fails catastrophically when dealing with complex symptoms, conditions that present atypically in your demographic, or healthcare systems operating under time pressure and algorithmic bias.

The healthcare advocates who achieve better outcomes understand that effective advocacy requires systematic preparation, strategic communication, and comprehensive health intelligence that most patients never develop. They use technology tools, research capabilities, and analytical frameworks to become informed partners in their healthcare rather than passive recipients of medical decisions.

This book provides the weapons you need for healthcare warfare—not against healthcare providers, but against the systems, biases, and limitations that prevent you from receiving the care you deserve. You'll learn to:

Family Health Intelligence. Build comprehensive family health intelligence that reveals the generational patterns and risk factors healthcare providers often miss.

Algorithmic Bias Recognition. Learn to recognize and counter the algorithmic bias built into the AI systems that increasingly shape diagnostic and treatment decisions.

Strategic Appointment Preparation. Prepare for medical appointments with the research, documentation, and organized evidence that commands respect from healthcare providers.

Lab and Data Interpretation. Interpret lab results and health data beyond the basic "normal" versus "abnormal" classifications to understand what the numbers actually mean for you.

Strategic Provider Communication. Communicate strategically with healthcare providers to secure the thorough evaluation and appropriate care you deserve.

Healthcare System Navigation. Navigate the full landscape of healthcare systems, insurance requirements, and administrative challenges that stand between you and good care.

Patient-Centered Provider Networks. Build networks of healthcare professionals who genuinely practice patient-centered care and value informed advocacy.

The goal isn't to replace medical expertise but to become an informed partner who can contribute meaningfully to health decisions, advocate effectively for appropriate care, and achieve health outcomes that passive patients rarely experience.

Your healthcare journey is too important to leave entirely in the hands of others. With AI as your strategic advisor and systematic advocacy as your approach, you can achieve the health outcomes you deserve while helping to transform healthcare for others facing similar challenges.

1

BUILDING YOUR AI HEALTHCARE COMMAND CENTER

From Patient to Strategic Health Advocate

The healthcare system was never designed with you in mind. If you're a woman, a person of color, someone with complex symptoms, or anyone who doesn't fit the narrow profile of a 70-kilogram white male, you've likely experienced medical dismissal, delayed diagnoses, or inadequate care. The statistics are sobering: women are 50% more likely to receive incorrect diagnoses for heart attacks, Black women are three to four times more likely to die from pregnancy-related complications, and patients with rare diseases wait an average of 7.6 years for accurate diagnosis.

But here's what the healthcare establishment doesn't want you to know: you can level the playing field using artificial intelligence as your strategic health advisor. This chapter will teach you to build your AI Healthcare Command Center—a comprehensive system that transforms you from a passive patient into an informed health advocate capable of navigating medical bias, tracking family health patterns, and communicating effectively with healthcare providers.

Setting Up Your AI Toolkit for Healthcare Advocacy and Research

Core AI Tools for Health Advocacy

Your AI Healthcare Command Center begins with selecting the right tools for medical research, symptom tracking, and health data analysis. Unlike generic AI applications, healthcare advocacy requires specialized approaches that prioritize accuracy, medical literature access, and bias-aware information gathering.

Primary Research Tools:

Womb WatchAI, ChatGPT-4, Claude for Medical Research Use these AI assistants to research symptoms, conditions, and treatment options before medical appointments. However, understand their limitations: they cannot provide medical advice and may reflect biases present in their training data. Always cross-reference AI-generated information with peer-reviewed medical sources.

> *Prompt Example: "Based on the symptoms of chronic fatigue, brain fog, and joint pain in a 35-year-old woman, what conditions should be investigated that are commonly missed or dismissed in women?"*

Perplexity AI for Medical Literature Search This tool excels at finding recent medical research and can cite specific studies. Use it to research cutting-edge treatments, clinical trials, and medical literature that your healthcare provider might not be aware of.

> *Prompt Example: "Find recent peer-reviewed studies on autoimmune conditions that present differently in women compared to men, focusing on research published in the last 3 years."*

Google Scholar Alerts Set up automated alerts for research related to your health conditions. This ensures you stay informed about new developments in treatment and diagnosis.

Health Data Organization Systems

Digital Health Record Creation

Most healthcare systems don't communicate effectively with each other, leaving you responsible for maintaining comprehensive health records. Create centralized digital system that includes:

Medication History. Document every medication with start dates, end dates, dosages, and any adverse reactions or side effects experienced.
Test Results. Keep all lab results with normal ranges specific to your demographics, noting any values that fall near the edges of "normal" even if not flagged.
Family Health History. Record every known condition across at least three generations, including ages of onset and outcomes.
Symptom Diary. Track all symptoms with dates, duration, triggers, and patterns over time. Include what makes symptoms better or worse.
Provider Directory. Maintain current contact information for every healthcare provider, including their specialty and the conditions they are managing for you.
Insurance Records. Document your coverage details, policy numbers, authorization requirements, and any claims that have been denied or disputed.

AI-Powered Symptom Tracking

Use AI to identify patterns in your symptoms that you might miss. Womb WatchAI and Expo Muscle Apps will offer Symptom Checkers that will help you articulate symptoms more precisely, but remember that these tools are for information gathering, not diagnosis.

Laboratory Result Analysis

AI can help you understand lab results beyond the basic "normal" or "abnormal" designation. Many lab values have different optimal ranges based on age, sex, ethnicity, and individual health goals. Use AI to research:

Optimal Ranges. Research the optimal ranges for your specific demographics rather than relying on the generic reference values printed on lab reports.
Result Trends. Examine trends in your results over time to identify shifts that may not trigger alerts on any single test but indicate meaningful change.
Borderline Result Questions. Develop questions to ask your doctor about borderline results that technically fall within "normal" but sit near the edges.
Additional Testing. Identify additional tests that might provide more information when initial results are unclear, borderline, or inconclusive.

Creating Secure Health Data Systems

Privacy and Security Considerations

Healthcare data is highly sensitive and protected by HIPAA regulations. When using AI tools for health research:

No Personal Identifiers. Never input personally identifiable information into AI systems, no matter how convenient it might feel.
General Descriptions. Use general descriptions rather than specific personal details when framing questions to AI tools.
Privacy Awareness. Understand that AI conversations may not be fully private and assume inputs could be reviewed, stored, or used to train future models.
Secure Storage. Keep detailed health records in secure, encrypted systems that are backed up and password protected.

Two-Factor Authentication. Use two-factor authentication on all health-related accounts to prevent unauthorized access to sensitive medical information.

Family Health History Database

Create a comprehensive family health database that goes beyond the basic questionnaire your doctor provides. This can be done using an excel spreadsheet and Include:

Detailed Conditions. Capture detailed health conditions for each family member, not just broad diagnostic categories.
Ages of Onset. Record the ages at which each condition first appeared, since early onset often signals higher genetic risk.
Environmental and Lifestyle Factors. Note the environmental factors and lifestyle patterns that may have influenced family health outcomes.
Occupational Exposures. Document occupational exposures to chemicals, radiation, or other workplace hazards across generations.
Geographic History. Record the geographic locations where family members lived, since regional exposures can influence disease patterns.
Reproductive History. Include pregnancy and birth complications that may reveal inherited reproductive health patterns.
Mental Health History. Track mental health history alongside physical conditions, since the two are often connected and frequently underreported.

Creating Strategic Frameworks for Medical Decision-Making and Appointment Preparation

Pre-Appointment Research Strategy

Symptom Documentation and Analysis

Before any medical appointment, use AI to help you organize and articulate your symptoms effectively. Healthcare providers often have limited time, so clarity and organization are crucial.

Symptom Preparation Framework:

Timeline Creation. Establish when symptoms started and how they have changed over time.
Pattern Recognition. Identify whether there are triggers, patterns, or cycles in how symptoms present.
Impact Assessment. Evaluate how symptoms affect daily life and function, including work, sleep, and relationships.
Previous Treatment. Summarize what has been tried and what the results were, including partial improvements and side effects.
Research Summary. Outline what conditions might explain your symptom cluster based on your own research.

> *AI Prompt for Symptom Organization: "Help me organize these symptoms into a clear, chronological summary for my doctor: [list symptoms]. Include questions I should ask about potential causes and diagnostic tests."*

Medical Literature Review

Use AI to research peer-reviewed studies related to your symptoms or conditions. Focus on:

Recent Research. Look for recent research that might not yet be standard practice but shows promising results.
Demographic-Specific Studies. Prioritize studies specific to your demographic in terms of age, sex, and ethnicity.
Alternative Diagnostic Approaches. Explore alternative diagnostic approaches that go beyond the default testing your provider may offer.
Expanded Treatment Options. Identify treatment options beyond what has been offered so you can ask informed questions.

Question Preparation

Develop strategic questions that demonstrate your informed participation in your healthcare. AI can help you formulate questions that encourage thorough evaluation rather than dismissal.

Examples of Strategic Questions:

Differential Diagnosis. "Given my symptom pattern, what differential diagnoses should we consider?"
Demographic Presentation. "Are there any conditions that present differently in [your demographic] that we should investigate?"
Commonly Missed Conditions. "What tests would help rule out conditions that are commonly missed in [your situation]?"
Family Member Framing. "If this were your family member, what would you want investigated?"

Diagnostic Test Strategy

Understanding Test Limitations

Many diagnostic tests have limitations that aren't always explained. Use AI to research:

Sensitivity and Specificity. Investigate the sensitivity and specificity of

proposed tests so you understand how reliable the results actually are.
False Negative Rates. Research false negative rates for your demographics, which can be significantly higher than average for some tests.
Alternative Tests. Consider alternative or additional tests that might be more appropriate for your situation.
Timing Considerations. Understand timing considerations for optimal test results, including hormonal cycle, time of day, or fasting requirements.

Advocating for Comprehensive Testing

Healthcare providers may order minimal testing due to cost concerns or bias. Research situations where more comprehensive testing is warranted:

Multi-Test Diagnoses. Identify conditions that require multiple tests for diagnosis rather than a single screening.
Commonly Skipped Tests. Know which tests are commonly skipped but clinically important for your profile.
Risk-Based Screening. Understand screening recommendations specific to your risk factors rather than population averages.
Second-Line Tests. Be prepared to request second-line tests when initial results are inconclusive.

Establishing Family Health Data Collection and Medical Record Analysis Systems

Comprehensive Family Health Mapping

Multi-Generational Health Analysis

Traditional family history collection is often superficial. Use AI to help you create a comprehensive multi-generational health analysis that can reveal patterns invisible to standard medical assessment.

Enhanced Family History Framework:

Condition Mapping. Document all health conditions across at least three generations to see the full landscape of inherited risk.
Age Pattern Analysis. Identify ages of onset for conditions, since early onset often indicates stronger genetic factors.
Gender Pattern Recognition. Note conditions that affect family members differently by gender, which can reveal hormonal or sex-linked patterns.
Environmental Factor Analysis. Consider geographic, occupational, and lifestyle factors that shaped family health outcomes.
Reproductive Health History. Include pregnancy complications, fertility issues, and hormonal conditions that often go unrecorded in standard histories.

> *AI Analysis Prompt: "Based on this family health history [provide anonymized data], what patterns suggest genetic predisposition, environmental factors, or conditions I should be monitored for? What questions should I ask my doctor about family history patterns?"*

Medical Record Analysis and Organization

Systematic Record Review

Most people don't maintain comprehensive medical records, making it difficult to identify patterns or advocate effectively. Use AI to help organize and analyze your medical history:

Medical Record Organization System:

Chronological Timeline. Build a chronological health timeline with major events, diagnoses, and procedures mapped in order.
Test Result Trends. Track test result trends over time rather than viewing each lab as an isolated snapshot.

Medication History and Response. Maintain a medication history with effectiveness and side effects noted for each.
Provider Notes. Keep copies of healthcare provider notes and recommendations so you can cross-reference what was said across visits.
Specialist Outcomes. Track specialist referrals and outcomes, including what was ruled in, ruled out, or left unresolved.

Identifying Gaps in Care

AI can help you identify potential gaps in your medical care by analyzing your health history against current screening guidelines and best practices.

> *Gap Analysis Prompt: "Based on my health history [provide relevant details], what screening tests, preventive care, or specialist consultations might be missing according to current medical guidelines for someone with my profile?"*

Developing Communication Strategies for Effective Doctor Interactions

Strategic Communication Frameworks

The SBAR Method for Healthcare Communication

Adapt the medical profession's SBAR (Situation, Background, Assessment, Recommendation) communication method for patient advocacy:

Situation: Current symptoms or health concerns **Background**: Relevant medical history and context **Assessment**: Your research and observations **Recommendation**: Specific requests for testing, referrals, or treatment

Overcoming Medical Bias Through Communication

Research shows that certain communication strategies can reduce the impact of medical bias:

Bring Documentation. Arrive with written symptom logs and research summaries that demonstrate the seriousness of your concerns.
Use Medical Terminology. Use medical terminology where appropriate to demonstrate your informed participation in the conversation.
Reference Specific Studies. Cite relevant research when appropriate to support your questions and requests.
Request Chart Documentation. Ask for notes about why tests or treatments are denied so there is a paper trail.
Bring an Advocate. A second person can witness interactions and provide support, which often changes the dynamic of the appointment.

Handling Dismissive Healthcare Providers

Recognition of Medical Gaslighting

Medical gaslighting occurs when healthcare providers dismiss, minimize, or misattribute patient symptoms. Common phrases that indicate potential bias:

"It's All in Your Head." This dismissal reframes physical symptoms as psychological without proper evaluation.
"You're Too Young for That Condition." This response treats age as a diagnostic shortcut instead of investigating symptoms.
"Just Stress or Anxiety." Attributing every symptom to stress or anxiety without investigation often masks conditions that require physical workup.
"Lose Weight and You'll Feel Better." This response uses weight to deflect from necessary diagnostic workup.

"Women Your Age Often Experience That." This framing treats disruptive symptoms as an expected consequence of being a woman of a certain age rather than something worth investigating.

Strategic Response Framework

When facing dismissive care, use these AI-developed response strategies:

Document Everything. Record dates, provider names, and exact phrases used during the appointment.
Request Specific Explanations. Ask the provider to explain the medical reasoning behind their assessment in concrete terms.
Cite Research. Point to recent studies showing the condition does occur in your demographic to push back on assumptions.
Request Chart Entry. Ask the provider to note in your chart that they are declining to test for a specific condition.
Escalate Appropriately. Know when to seek second opinions or file complaints rather than continuing in a dismissive relationship.

Building Confidence to Seek Second Opinions and Advocate for Yourself

Second Opinion Strategy

When to Seek Second Opinions

Use AI to research situations where second opinions are medically advisable:

Rare or Complex Diagnoses. Rare or complex diagnoses benefit from additional expert perspectives because no single provider sees enough cases to know every nuance.

Major Treatment Decisions. Major treatment decisions deserve a second opinion before you commit to an irreversible course of action.
Unexplained Persistent Symptoms. When symptoms persist without explanation, another clinician may see what the first one missed.
Pre-Surgical Evaluation. Before surgical procedures, confirm that the surgery is necessary and appropriately matched to your condition.
Dismissive Encounters. When you feel dismissed or unheard, a second opinion can restore confidence and often changes the diagnosis entirely.

How to Obtain Effective Second Opinions

Choose Different Healthcare Systems. Avoid providers within the same network, since providers in the same system often share notes and assumptions.
Seek Specialists. Ensure the second opinion comes from relevant expertise in the condition being evaluated.
Provide Complete Information. Share all records and test results so the second provider works from the same evidence base.
Ask Specific Questions. Focus on areas where you need clarity rather than asking for a general review.
Consider Academic Medical Centers. Teaching hospitals often provide comprehensive evaluation and are more likely to consider rare or complex presentations.

Building Long-Term Health Advocacy Skills

Developing Medical Literacy

Use AI as a learning tool to gradually build your understanding of medical concepts, terminology, and systems. Focus on:

Understanding Your Conditions. Deepen your understanding of your specific health conditions over time so you can engage as a partner rather than a passive recipient of information.

Interpreting Tests and Procedures. Learn to interpret common tests and procedures so you can spot issues before your provider flags them.
Recognizing Quality Care. Develop the ability to recognize quality healthcare practices and the red flags that indicate substandard care.
Knowing Your Rights. Understand your rights as a patient, including access to records, informed consent, and second-opinion rights.

Creating Support Networks

AI can help you find and connect with:

Patient Advocacy Organizations. Patient advocacy organizations can connect you with resources, research, and community that individual advocacy cannot.
Condition-Specific Support Groups. Support groups for your specific conditions provide both emotional support and practical information from people further along in the journey.
Patient-Centered Providers. Identify healthcare providers who practice patient-centered care and are a better fit for informed advocates.
Legal Resources. Know the legal resources available for medical malpractice or discrimination should the need arise.

Measuring Success in Healthcare Advocacy

Key Performance Indicators for Health Advocacy

Track your progress in becoming an effective health advocate:

Time to Accurate Diagnosis. Reduced time to accurate diagnosis is one of the strongest indicators that your advocacy approach is working.
Interaction Satisfaction. Increased satisfaction with healthcare interactions reflects improved communication and mutual respect with providers.

Health Outcomes. Better health outcomes and symptom management signal that advocacy is translating into real clinical benefit.
Communication Quality. Improved communication with healthcare providers means your concerns are being heard and documented.
Decision-Making Confidence. Greater confidence in medical decision-making reflects the growing medical literacy you've built over time.

Continuous Improvement

Use AI to regularly assess and improve your health advocacy approach:

Interaction Analysis. Analyze successful and unsuccessful healthcare interactions to learn what approaches produce the best outcomes.
Ongoing Research. Research new developments in your health conditions so your knowledge remains current.
Strategy Updates. Update your health advocacy strategies based on outcomes and what you've learned works for you.
Knowledge Sharing. Share knowledge with others facing similar challenges to strengthen the broader advocacy community.

Your Healthcare Command Center Foundation

Building your AI Healthcare Command Center is not about replacing medical professionals—it's about becoming an informed partner in your healthcare. By systematically organizing your health data, researching your conditions, and communicating strategically with providers, you transform from a passive patient into an active health advocate.

The tools and frameworks outlined in this chapter provide the foundation for everything that follows in this book. As you progress through subsequent chapters, you'll learn to identify and combat algorithmic bias, master family health intelligence, and build comprehensive health advocacy skills that can literally save your life.

Remember: your health is too important to leave entirely in the hands of a biased healthcare system. With AI as your strategic advisor and these systematic approaches as your guide, you can navigate healthcare challenges with confidence and achieve better health outcomes for yourself and your family.

The war room you're building isn't just about fighting for better healthcare—it's about claiming your rightful role as the primary advocate for your own health and wellbeing. In the following chapters, we'll weaponize these foundations to combat specific challenges within the healthcare system and beyond.

Exercise 1.1 – Your Personal Health Journal

Take 10 minutes to write down every health concern you currently have, every medication you take, every ongoing symptom, and every question you've wanted to ask a doctor but haven't. Don't filter yourself. This is the foundation of your Command Center.

Reflection: *Which of these concerns have you been dismissing as "not important enough to bring up"? Why?*

Exercise 1.2 – Your AI Tool Inventory

List the AI tools you already have access to (Rhythm by Womb WatchAI, ChatGPT, Claude, Perplexity, Womb WatchAI, etc.) and what you've used them for in the past. Now write down three specific health questions you could ask an AI tool this week to start practicing.

Reflection: *What is one question you've been afraid to research because you didn't want to know the answer?*

2

UNDERSTANDING AND EXPOSING ALGORITHMIC BIAS IN HEALTHCARE

The Hidden Algorithms Controlling Your Care

Every time you interact with the healthcare system, artificial intelligence systems are making decisions about your care—often without your knowledge or consent. From the moment you schedule an appointment to the treatment recommendations your doctor receives, algorithms trained on biased data are influencing medical decisions that directly impact your health and wellbeing.

These AI systems aren't neutral. They carry forward decades of medical research that systematically excluded women, minorities, and diverse populations. The result is a healthcare AI ecosystem that perpetuates and amplifies existing disparities, making it even harder for marginalized groups to receive appropriate care.

This chapter will teach you to identify, understand, and counter algorithmic bias in healthcare. You'll learn to recognize when AI systems are working against you, how to research unbiased medical information, and strategies to advocate for care that considers your individual needs rather than biased algorithmic assumptions.

How AI Systems in Healthcare Perpetuate Bias Against Women and Minorities

The Foundation of Biased Healthcare AI

Historical Medical Research Bias

Healthcare AI systems are trained on decades of medical research that was fundamentally flawed from the start. Until the 1993 NIH Revitalization Act, medical research routinely excluded women from clinical trials under the assumption that female hormones would "complicate" results. This exclusion wasn't just oversight—it was institutionalized practice that created massive gaps in medical knowledge.

The impact compounds when this biased research becomes training data for AI systems:

Drug Dosing Algorithms. Drug dosing algorithms are often based on male metabolism and routinely lead to misdosing women as a result.
Diagnostic Criteria. Diagnostic criteria miss female presentations of disease because the reference symptoms were defined from male subjects.
Risk Assessment Tools. Risk assessment tools underestimate women's health risks across multiple categories including cardiovascular disease.
Treatment Protocols. Treatment protocols assume male physiology as the standard and apply those assumptions uniformly.

Racial and Ethnic Bias in Medical AI

The problem extends beyond gender. Medical AI systems trained primarily on data from white populations consistently misdiagnose and undertreat patients of color:

Pulse Oximeters. Pulse oximeters overestimate blood oxygen levels in patients with darker skin, leading to missed cases of dangerously low oxygen.
Pain Assessment Algorithms. Pain assessment algorithms systematically underestimate pain in Black patients, resulting in undertreatment.
Kidney Function Calculators. Kidney function calculators historically used race as a variable, leading to delayed treatment for Black patients with declining kidney function.
Dermatology AI Systems. Dermatology AI systems fail to recognize skin conditions on darker skin tones because the training images were disproportionately light-skinned.

Current Healthcare AI Systems and Their Biases

Electronic Health Record (EHR) Decision Support

Most healthcare providers use EHR systems with built-in decision support algorithms. These systems:

Demographic-Weighted Flags. They flag certain symptoms as more or less concerning based on patient demographics rather than clinical presentation alone.
Divergent Treatment Pathways. They suggest different treatment pathways based on biased risk calculations built from incomplete data.
Provider Alerts and Nudges. They influence provider behavior through alerts and recommendations that providers may follow without questioning the underlying logic.

Opaque Decision Logic. They often lack transparency about how decisions are made, leaving both patients and providers unable to examine the reasoning.

Diagnostic Imaging AI

AI systems used to interpret medical images carry significant bias:

Chest X-ray Algorithms. Chest X-ray algorithms trained primarily on male patients miss female-specific presentations of pulmonary and cardiac conditions.

Mammography AI. Mammography AI systems show reduced accuracy for women with dense breast tissue, which is more common in women of color.

Cardiac Imaging AI. Cardiac imaging AI misses heart disease patterns that are more common in women and presents them as normal studies.

Risk Prediction Algorithms

Healthcare systems use AI to predict which patients need more intensive care or are at risk for complications. These algorithms consistently show bias:

Sepsis Prediction. Sepsis prediction algorithms delay treatment for women and minorities whose presentations don't match the model's expectations.

Readmission Risk Tools. Readmission risk tools underestimate risk for marginalized populations who then receive less post-discharge support.

Pain Prediction Algorithms. Pain prediction algorithms assume certain groups have higher pain tolerance, leading to systematic undertreatment.

Identifying Biased Algorithms in Diagnostic Tools and Treatment Recommendations

Red Flags of Algorithmic Bias in Healthcare

Demographic-Based Assumptions

Watch for situations where your healthcare provider makes assumptions based on demographic characteristics rather than individual symptoms:

Age-Based Dismissal. Age-based dismissal of symptoms such as "you're too young for that condition" signals that a demographic shortcut is replacing clinical investigation.

Gender-Based Assumptions. Gender-based assumptions about pain tolerance or symptom presentation often lead to minimization of real physical problems.

Racial or Ethnic Assumptions. Racial or ethnic assumptions about disease risk or pain perception distort both diagnosis and treatment.

Weight-Based Dismissal. Weight-based dismissal of symptoms without proper investigation is one of the most common forms of bias women encounter.

Pattern Recognition of Biased Responses

Use AI to help identify patterns that suggest algorithmic bias is influencing your care:

> *AI Analysis Prompt: "Based on these interactions with healthcare providers [describe situations], help me identify potential patterns of bias. What questions should I ask to determine if algorithmic decision support is influencing my care?"*

Standard Treatment Protocols That May Not Fit

Many healthcare algorithms assume one-size-fits-all solutions that may not be appropriate for diverse populations:

Uniform Medication Dosing. Medication dosing that doesn't account for genetic variations in drug metabolism can lead to under- or over-dosing in specific populations.
Narrow Diagnostic Criteria. Diagnostic criteria miss atypical presentations common in certain demographics, delaying correct diagnosis.
Standardized Treatment Timelines. Treatment timelines that don't consider different healing patterns across populations can mislead providers about treatment success.

Investigating Algorithmic Influence in Your Care

Questions to Ask Healthcare Providers

Develop specific questions that can help reveal whether algorithmic bias is affecting your care:

Decision Support Tools. "What clinical decision support tools or algorithms influenced this recommendation?"
Demographic Accounting. "How does this diagnostic criteria account for differences in symptom presentation across demographics?"
Training Data Composition. "What data was this risk assessment tool trained on, and does it include people like me?"
Alternative Approaches. "Are there alternative diagnostic approaches that might be more appropriate for my demographic?"
Disparity Awareness. "Can you explain how this algorithm accounts for known disparities in healthcare?"

Researching Healthcare AI Systems

Use AI research tools to investigate the decision support systems your healthcare providers might be using:

> *Research Prompt: "Find information about common clinical decision support algorithms used in [specific medical specialty]. What are known bias issues with these systems, and what questions should patients ask about algorithmic decision-making?"*

Documentation and Advocacy

When you suspect algorithmic bias is affecting your care:

Document Specific Instances. Document specific instances where demographic assumptions influenced treatment decisions.
Request Algorithm Information. Request information about what algorithms or decision support tools were used in your care.
Ask for Alternatives. Ask for alternative approaches that don't rely on potentially biased algorithms.
Seek Second Opinions. Seek second opinions from providers who may use different systems or approaches to evaluation.

Understanding the Male Default in Medical Research and AI Training Data

The Male Default Problem

Historical Research Exclusion

For decades, medical research operated under the "male default" assumption—that male bodies represented the standard human experience and that findings could be extrapolated to women. This created fundamental gaps in medical knowledge:

Cardiovascular Research. Cardiovascular disease research focused on male presentations, missing female-specific symptoms and patterns.
Drug Trials. Drug trials excluded women of childbearing age, leading to inappropriate dosing and unknown side-effect profiles for women.
Pain Research. Pain research used primarily male subjects, creating pain assessment tools that minimize female pain experiences.
Mental Health Research. Mental health research often ignored hormonal influences on conditions like depression and anxiety.

How AI Amplifies the Male Default

When AI systems are trained on this biased historical data, they don't just preserve bias—they amplify it:

Prioritization of Male Presentations. Algorithms learn to prioritize male symptom presentations as "typical" in ways that reinforce the original bias.
Classification of Female Symptoms. Female symptoms get classified as "atypical" or less concerning, which reduces urgency in care pathways.
Default Treatment Recommendations. Treatment recommendations default to protocols designed for male physiology without flagging the mismatch.
Underestimated Risk. Risk assessments underestimate female health risks in many conditions, leading to undertreatment and late intervention.

Specific Examples of Male Default Bias in Healthcare AI

Cardiovascular Disease

Heart disease AI systems trained primarily on male data consistently miss female presentations:

Heart Attack Misdiagnosis. Women are 50% more likely to receive misdiagnosis for heart attacks because the criteria were built around male presentations.
Atypical Symptom Labeling. Female heart attack symptoms such as fatigue, shortness of breath, and nausea are classified as "atypical" despite being typical for women.
Stress Testing Algorithms. Stress testing algorithms show reduced accuracy for women, producing more false reassurance.
Cardiac Risk Calculators. Cardiac risk calculators underestimate risk for younger women and delay preventive intervention.

Pain Assessment and Management

Pain management algorithms consistently underestimate and undertreat pain in women:

Male-Derived Pain Scales. Pain scales developed using male subjects don't accurately capture female pain experiences.
Drug-Seeking Assumptions. Algorithms assume women are more likely to be "drug-seeking" or exaggerating pain, which biases clinical responses.
Psychological Reclassification. Chronic pain conditions more common in women are often classified as psychological rather than physical.

Autoimmune Conditions

Despite being significantly more common in women, autoimmune disease diagnostics show persistent bias:

Delayed Recognition. Diagnostic algorithms delay recognition of autoimmune conditions in women, extending time to diagnosis by years.
Misattribution of Early Symptoms. Early symptoms are often attributed to stress, anxiety, or hormonal issues rather than autoimmune disease.
Male-Dominated Training Data. AI systems trained on male-dominated research miss female-specific presentations of autoimmune illness.

Countering the Male Default in Your Healthcare

Research Female-Specific Presentations

Use AI to research how conditions present differently in women compared to the standard (male) descriptions:

> *Research Prompt: "How does [specific condition] present differently in women compared to men? What symptoms or presentations are commonly missed when using male-default diagnostic criteria?"*

Advocate for Gender-Specific Protocols

When discussing symptoms or treatment with healthcare providers:

Ask About Female Presentations. Specifically ask about female presentations of your condition and how they may differ from the default criteria.
Request Hormonal Consideration. Request consideration of hormonal influences on your symptoms, including menstrual cycle, pregnancy history, and menopause.
Ask About Female Trial Inclusion. Ask whether treatment protocols have been tested in women and how outcomes compared to male subjects.
Inquire About Dosing Adjustments. Inquire about dosing adjustments for female physiology rather than accepting default doses.

Seek Female-Focused Healthcare Providers

Research healthcare providers and systems that specialize in addressing gender disparities:

Women's Health Specialists. Women's health specialists understand gender-specific presentations that general providers often miss.
Bias-Aware Systems. Seek out healthcare systems with protocols designed to address bias and close disparity gaps.
Disparity-Informed Providers. Prioritize providers who stay current with research on health disparities and apply it in their practice.

Recognizing When Algorithmic Bias Affects Your Care

Warning Signs of Algorithmic Bias

Immediate Red Flags

Learn to recognize situations where algorithmic bias may be influencing your care:

Rapid Dismissal. Your symptoms are quickly attributed to stress, anxiety, or weight without thorough investigation of physical causes.
Demographic Assumptions. Treatment recommendations seem based on your age, gender, or race rather than individual symptoms.
Standard Protocol Rigidity. Providers seem unwilling to consider alternative approaches or protocols even when the standard approach isn't producing results.
Pain Minimization. Your pain reports are consistently questioned or minimized despite their impact on daily life.

Delayed Referrals. Specialist referrals are delayed or denied despite persistent symptoms that warrant evaluation.

Systemic Patterns to Watch For

Gender-Based Dismissal Patterns:

Hormonal or Emotional Attribution. Female symptoms are attributed to hormones, stress, or emotional issues without corresponding physical workup.

Pain Complaint Minimization. Pain complaints are treated as exaggeration or attention-seeking rather than legitimate clinical data.

Cluster Dismissal. Complex symptom clusters are dismissed as "normal female experiences" without investigation.

Delayed Female-Specific Diagnosis. Delayed diagnosis occurs for conditions that present differently in women due to reliance on male-default criteria.

Age-Based Bias Patterns:

Too Young Dismissal. Young patients are told they're "too young" for certain conditions despite credible symptoms.

Aging Attribution. Older patients have symptoms attributed solely to aging rather than treatable conditions.

Menopause Attribution. Middle-aged women have symptoms dismissed as menopause-related when the underlying cause is something else.

Weight-Based Bias Patterns:

Blanket Weight Attribution. All symptoms are attributed to weight without investigation of other causes.

Weight-Gated Testing. Diagnostic testing is delayed until weight loss is achieved, which can miss time-sensitive conditions.

Weight-Only Recommendations. Treatment recommendations focus solely on weight management instead of addressing the presenting symptoms directly.

Using AI to Identify Bias in Your Healthcare Experience

Pattern Analysis

Use AI to analyze your healthcare experiences for potential bias patterns:

> *Bias Detection Prompt: "Analyze these healthcare interactions for potential bias: [describe appointments, diagnoses, treatment recommendations]. What patterns suggest algorithmic or provider bias, and what questions should I ask to address these concerns?"*

Alternative Research Strategies

When you suspect bias is affecting your care, use AI to research alternative approaches:

> *Alternative Research Prompt: "Find recent research on [your condition] that specifically addresses disparities in diagnosis and treatment across gender/racial/age groups. What alternative diagnostic approaches or treatment protocols show better outcomes for people like me?"*

Documentation for Advocacy

Create systematic documentation of potential bias incidents:

Provider Statements. Record the date, provider, and specific statements made during each appointment.
Testing Decisions. Note the diagnostic tests ordered or refused and the reasoning given.
Treatment Justification. Document treatment recommendations and their stated justification.

Contradicting Research. Keep copies of your research findings that contradict provider assumptions.
Outcome Tracking. Track the outcomes of different approaches to build evidence for future advocacy.

Tools to Research Unbiased Medical Information and Alternative Perspectives

Identifying High-Quality, Bias-Aware Medical Sources

Academic and Research Institutions

Focus on sources that actively address healthcare disparities:

Diversity-Focused Institutions. Research from institutions with diversity and inclusion focus tends to address the blind spots of mainstream research.
Disparity-Specific Studies. Studies that specifically examine health disparities provide the most directly applicable evidence for bias-resistant care.
Inclusive Meta-Analyses. Meta-analyses that include diverse populations offer a broader view than single-study findings from narrow populations.
International Research. Research from countries with different healthcare approaches can reveal assumptions baked into US-centric medicine.

Specialized Organizations

Leverage organizations dedicated to addressing healthcare bias:

American Medical Women's Association (AMWA). The American Medical Women's Association focuses on advancing women in medicine and addressing gender-based health disparities.

National Medical Association. The National Medical Association addresses racial health disparities and centers the concerns of Black physicians and patients.
Society for Women's Health Research. The Society for Women's Health Research promotes research into sex differences and women's health conditions.
Office of Research on Women's Health (NIH). The Office of Research on Women's Health at NIH funds and coordinates research on women's health across federal agencies.

International Research Sources

Look beyond US-based research for alternative perspectives:

European Research. European medical research often includes different population bases and regulatory frameworks.
Universal Healthcare Studies. Studies from countries with universal healthcare systems can reveal outcomes less shaped by insurance access.
Regional Women's Health Approaches. Research from regions with different approaches to women's health offers valuable alternative models.
International Guidelines. International guidelines may differ from US standards and can inform conversations with your providers.

AI-Powered Research Strategies

Bias-Aware Research Prompts

Use specific prompts to find research that addresses bias and disparities:

> *Disparity Research Prompt: "Find recent peer-reviewed studies on [condition] that specifically examine differences in presentation, diagnosis, or treatment across gender, racial, or ethnic groups. Focus on research published in the last 5 years that addresses healthcare disparities."*

Alternative Protocol Prompt: "Research alternative diagnostic or treatment approaches for [condition] that have shown better outcomes for [your demographic group]. Include international research and non-standard protocols that address known biases in typical care."

Cross-Referencing and Validation

Develop systematic approaches to validate medical information:

Multiple Source Verification. Cross-reference findings across different types of sources to confirm consistency.
Demographic-Specific Research. Look for studies that include people like you rather than accepting findings from unrepresentative samples.
Recent Research Priority. Focus on research from the last 3–5 years that may address known biases and reflect current understanding.
Methodology Assessment. Evaluate research methodology for inclusion and bias considerations before accepting conclusions.

Building Alternative Information Networks

Patient Advocacy Organizations

Connect with organizations focused on your specific conditions or demographic:

Disease-Specific Organizations. Disease-specific organizations with patient advocacy focus often have the most current information on diagnosis and treatment options.
Disparity-Focused Groups. Organizations addressing healthcare disparities can connect you with resources that mainstream channels overlook.
Patient-Led Research. Patient-led research initiatives often identify issues years before mainstream medicine acknowledges them.

Shared-Experience Support Groups. Support groups with shared experiences can offer practical insight into what approaches actually work.

Healthcare Providers with Bias Awareness

Research and identify healthcare providers who demonstrate awareness of bias issues:

Bias-Trained Providers. Providers who participate in bias training or disparity research are more likely to recognize and address it in practice.
Anti-Bias Protocols. Healthcare systems with explicit anti-bias protocols build accountability into their care delivery.
Disparity-Citing Clinicians. Providers who cite research on healthcare disparities have already demonstrated engagement with the issue.
Advocates for Underserved Populations. Medical professionals who advocate for underserved populations often bring that awareness into individual patient care.

Alternative and Integrative Approaches

Research evidence-based alternative approaches that may address gaps in conventional care:

Integrative Medicine. Integrative medicine approaches with research backing can complement conventional care without replacing it.
Traditional Medicine Practices. Traditional medicine practices with documented efficacy offer options that have been refined over generations.
Lifestyle and Environmental Interventions. Lifestyle and environmental interventions can address root causes that medication alone cannot.
Functional Medicine. Functional medicine approaches that address root causes can provide frameworks for chronic conditions that conventional care struggles with.

Advanced Strategies for Countering Algorithmic Bias

Preparing for Bias-Aware Healthcare Encounters

Pre-Appointment Research Protocol

Develop a systematic approach to pre-appointment preparation that accounts for potential bias:

Demographic-Specific Research. Research how your condition presents in people with your demographic characteristics before the appointment.
Alternative Diagnostic Criteria. Identify diagnostic approaches that may be more appropriate for your situation than the defaults.
Bias Documentation. Prepare documentation of known biases related to your condition and demographic so you can reference it in discussion.
Question Development. Develop specific questions that address potential bias in care and invite the provider to engage with it directly.

Communication Strategies for Bias Resistance

Evidence-Based Advocacy:

Cite Disparity Research. Cite specific research that addresses disparities in your condition to ground your concerns in evidence.
Reference Alternative Criteria. Reference alternative diagnostic criteria when appropriate rather than accepting the default framework.
Provide Pattern Documentation. Provide documentation of symptom patterns that don't fit standard algorithms.
Request Algorithmic Explanation. Request explanation of algorithmic recommendations and the basis on which they were made.

Collaborative Language:

Partner Positioning. Position yourself as a research partner rather than a passive patient.
Medical Terminology. Use medical terminology appropriately to demonstrate knowledge and shift the dynamic of the interaction.
Collaborative Framing. Frame requests as collaborative problem-solving rather than confrontational challenges.
Acknowledge Expertise While Asserting Needs. Acknowledge provider expertise while asserting your individual needs so both can coexist in the conversation.

Long-Term Strategies for Bias-Resistant Healthcare

Building Your Healthcare Team

Systematically identify and work with providers who demonstrate bias awareness:

Provider Research. Research providers' publications or statements on healthcare disparities before choosing them.
Initial Consultation Questions. Ask specific questions about bias awareness during initial consultations to assess fit.
Openness to Alternatives. Evaluate providers' willingness to consider alternative approaches rather than defaulting to standard protocols.
Relationship Building. Build relationships with providers who acknowledge and address bias over time.

Creating Accountability Systems

Develop systems to hold healthcare providers accountable for bias-free care:

Detailed Documentation. Document all interactions with detailed notes so patterns can be identified over time.

Written Decision Explanations. Request written explanations for diagnostic or treatment decisions whenever possible.
Second Opinions. Ask for second opinions when bias is suspected rather than continuing in a questionable relationship.
Portal Communication. Use patient portal systems to maintain written communication records that cannot be disputed later.

Advocacy Beyond Personal Care

Use your experience to advocate for broader systemic change:

Reporting Bias Incidents. Report bias incidents to appropriate oversight bodies so the system can track and respond to patterns.
Patient Advisory Participation. Participate in patient advisory groups or healthcare system committees where policy is shaped.
Experience Sharing. Share experiences with advocacy organizations that amplify individual stories into systemic pressure.
Supporting Disparity Research. Support research that addresses healthcare disparities through participation, donation, or advocacy.

Becoming Bias-Resistant in Healthcare

Understanding and exposing algorithmic bias in healthcare isn't just about getting better care for yourself—it's about challenging systems that perpetuate health disparities for millions of people. By learning to recognize bias, research alternatives, and advocate effectively, you become part of the solution to healthcare inequality.

The strategies outlined in this chapter provide you with tools to identify when algorithms are working against you and methods to counter that bias through informed advocacy. As healthcare becomes increasingly dependent on AI systems, your ability to recognize and challenge bias becomes even more critical.

Remember that algorithmic bias in healthcare isn't a bug—it's a feature of systems built on biased data and assumptions. Changing these systems requires patients who understand the problem and are equipped to advocate for bias-free care. Your healthcare command center now includes the intelligence gathering and analytical tools necessary to identify bias and fight for equitable treatment.

In the next chapter, we'll build on this foundation to explore how AI can help you master family health history intelligence, identifying patterns that biased healthcare systems often miss or dismiss. The combination of bias awareness and comprehensive family health analysis creates a powerful advocacy framework that can reveal health risks and opportunities that traditional medicine overlooks.

Exercise 2.1 – Your Bias Story

Describe a time when you felt dismissed, misdiagnosed, or rushed through a medical appointment. Write the full story — what you said, what the provider said, how you felt. Don't worry about being "fair" to the provider. This is your experience.

Reflection: Looking back, what would you do differently today with what you've learned in this chapter?

Exercise 2.2 – Your Demographic Risk Profile

Write down your age, sex, ethnicity, and any other demographic factors that might affect how healthcare providers or AI systems assess you. Then research (or use AI to research) which conditions are commonly misdiagnosed in people with your profile.

___

___

___

___

___

___

___

___

___

___

___

___

Reflection: *What conditions should you proactively ask about at your next appointment based on your demographic risk profile?*

3

MASTERING FAMILY HEALTH HISTORY INTELLIGENCE

Beyond "Runs in the Family"

When doctors tell you a condition "runs in your family," they're often using this phrase as a conversation stopper rather than a starting point for investigation. The standard family history questionnaire you fill out at medical appointments barely scratches the surface of what your family's health patterns can reveal about your own risks, optimal treatments, and prevention strategies.

Healthcare providers typically collect family history in the most superficial way possible: major diseases in immediate relatives, ages of death, and perhaps a few details about grandparents. This approach misses crucial patterns that could transform your healthcare. It ignores environmental factors, timing patterns, gender-specific presentations, and the complex interplay between genetics, lifestyle, and environmental exposures that actually determine health outcomes.

This chapter will teach you to become a family health intelligence analyst, using AI tools to identify patterns that healthcare systems miss, understand the true meaning behind familial health trends, and leverage this intelligence for better prevention, earlier detection, and more personalized treatment approaches.

AI-Powered Family Health Pattern Analysis and Genetic Risk Assessment

Moving Beyond Basic Family History

The Limitations of Standard Medical Family History

Traditional family history collection in healthcare settings is designed for speed and convenience, not insight. The typical questionnaire asks about:

Immediate Family Diseases. The standard form captures major diseases in parents and siblings but little else.
Ages of Death. The form asks for ages of death for immediate relatives without context about circumstances or causes.
Limited Grandparent Questions. Only a few superficial questions about grandparents are typically included.
Yes/No Simplification. The form reduces complex family health history to simple yes/no answers about common conditions.

This approach misses critical information that could dramatically impact your health strategy:

Shared Environmental Exposures. Environmental exposures that affected multiple family members are rarely captured in standard forms.
Timing Patterns. Timing patterns that reveal genetic versus environmental influences are invisible without detailed onset data.
Gender-Specific Presentations. Gender-specific presentations that

might predict your risk are lost when forms treat all relatives the same.
Protective Factor Variations. Protective factors that some family members had but others didn't are rarely examined in medical settings.
Subclinical Conditions. Subclinical conditions that never received formal diagnosis are missing entirely from clinical family histories.

Building Comprehensive Family Health Intelligence

Use AI to help you develop a far more sophisticated understanding of your family health patterns:

> *Comprehensive Analysis Prompt: "Help me analyze this family health information [provide anonymized data] for patterns that might indicate: genetic predisposition, environmental factors, timing correlations, gender-specific presentations, and protective factors. What questions should I research about each pattern identified?"*

Systematic Family Health Data Collection

Multi-Generational Health Mapping Framework

Create a comprehensive family health database that goes far beyond what any medical office collects:

Immediate Family (Parents, Siblings, Children):

Complete Diagnoses with Onset. Document complete medical diagnoses with ages of onset for each condition.
Pre-Diagnosis Symptom Patterns. Capture symptom patterns that preceded formal diagnoses, which often reveal inherited presentations.
Environmental Exposures. Record environmental exposures including occupational, geographic, and lifestyle factors.
Reproductive History. Include reproductive history including pregnancy complications, fertility issues, and hormonal conditions.

Treatment Response Patterns. Document response patterns to treatments and medications that may predict your own response.
Lifestyle Factors. Include lifestyle factors such as diet, exercise, and stress levels that influence health outcomes.
Mental Health History. Capture mental health history including undiagnosed depression or anxiety that may run in the family.

Extended Family (Grandparents, Aunts, Uncles, Cousins):

Conditions and Onset Ages. Record major health conditions and ages of onset for each extended family member.
Causes and Circumstances of Death. Document causes of death and the circumstances surrounding them when known.
Geographic Locations. Note the geographic locations where they lived and worked across their lifetimes.
Known Environmental Exposures. Capture any known environmental exposures from their homes, workplaces, or communities.
Lifestyle and Socioeconomic Factors. Record lifestyle patterns and socioeconomic factors that shaped their health outcomes.
Longevity Patterns. Note any patterns of early death or unusual longevity that may indicate genetic or environmental influences.

Historical Context Research:

Location-Based Hazards. Research environmental hazards in locations where family lived during key periods.
Era-Specific Occupational Exposures. Investigate occupational exposures common during their working years that may not be obvious today.
Historical Health Events. Document historical health events such as epidemics or environmental disasters that affected family members.
Cultural and Dietary Patterns. Note cultural and dietary patterns that might influence health across generations.

Healthcare Access Factors. Record economic factors that affected healthcare access and influenced when conditions were diagnosed or treated.

AI-Enhanced Pattern Recognition

Identifying Genetic Versus Environmental Influences

Use AI to help distinguish between genetic predisposition and environmental factors:

> *Pattern Discrimination Prompt: "Analyze this family health data to help distinguish between genetic predisposition and environmental factors: [provide data]. What patterns suggest genetic influence versus shared environmental exposures? What additional information would help clarify these distinctions?"*

Timing Pattern Analysis

Look for timing patterns that reveal important health intelligence:

Same-Age Condition Clusters. Identify conditions that appear at similar ages across family members, which may indicate genetic timing.
Life-Event Health Clusters. Notice health problems that cluster around major life events such as childbirth, job changes, or loss.
Seasonal or Cyclical Patterns. Watch for seasonal or cyclical patterns in family health issues that may point to environmental triggers.
Generational Differences. Look for generational differences that might indicate environmental changes across time periods.

Gender-Specific Pattern Recognition

Many health conditions present differently or have different risk factors based on gender:

Gender-Differential Autoimmune Conditions. Track autoimmune conditions that affect women differently than men in your family.

Gender-Based Cardiovascular Patterns. Examine cardiovascular disease patterns that vary by gender across family members.
Maternal vs. Paternal Cancer Risks. Identify cancer risks that follow maternal versus paternal lines to clarify your inherited risk.
Hormonal Condition Influences. Consider hormonal influences on conditions like depression or diabetes that may present differently by sex.

Tracking Hereditary Conditions and Environmental Health Factors Across Generations

Understanding True Hereditary Risk

Beyond Simple Genetic Determinism

The phrase "genetic predisposition" is often misunderstood. Most conditions involve complex interactions between genetics, environment, and lifestyle. Use AI to help understand what family health patterns actually mean:

> *Risk Assessment Prompt: "Based on this family health pattern [specific condition appearing in multiple relatives], what does current research say about genetic versus environmental risk factors? What preventive measures have shown effectiveness for people with this family history?"*

Penetrance and Expression Patterns

Not everyone with genetic risk develops the condition. Analyze your family patterns to understand:

Penetrance Rate. Estimate what percentage of at-risk family members actually developed the condition.

Protective Factors. Identify environmental or lifestyle factors that seemed protective for unaffected family members.
Onset Age Patterns. Map age patterns for condition onset to understand when you might be most at risk.
Severity Variations. Document severity variations among affected family members, since expression often varies even with the same risk.

Environmental Health Factor Analysis

Occupational and Geographic Clustering

Look for environmental patterns that might explain family health clusters:

Occupational Exposure Analysis:

Shared Industries. Identify industries where multiple family members worked, which may reveal shared occupational risks.
Workplace Hazards. Research common workplace chemicals or hazards specific to those industries and eras.
Employment–Health Timing. Examine timing correlation between employment and health issues to pinpoint causal links.
Regional Occupational Patterns. Look for regional occupational health patterns that affected communities where family members worked.

Geographic Health Mapping:

Critical-Period Locations. Map locations where family members lived during critical periods of development and exposure.
Area-Specific Hazards. Research environmental hazards specific to those areas during the years family members lived there.
Water, Air, and Industrial Contamination. Investigate water quality,

air pollution, or industrial contamination that may have affected the community.

Agricultural Chemical Exposures. Consider agricultural chemical exposures in rural areas where family members lived or worked.

> *Environmental Analysis Prompt: "Help me analyze potential environmental health factors for my family based on this information: [geographic and occupational data]. What environmental hazards were common in these locations during these time periods, and what health conditions are associated with these exposures?"*

Lifestyle and Cultural Pattern Analysis

Examine lifestyle patterns that might influence family health:

Dietary Patterns. Examine dietary patterns and food traditions that shaped multiple generations.

Physical Activity. Note physical activity levels and types that characterized healthy or unhealthy family members.

Stress Management. Record stress management approaches that family members used effectively or poorly.

Healthcare Utilization. Document healthcare utilization patterns including whether family members sought or avoided care.

Social and Economic Factors. Consider social and economic factors affecting health across family members and generations.

Generational Health Trend Analysis

Tracking Changes Across Generations

Use AI to identify how health patterns change across generations in your family:

> *Generational Analysis Prompt: "Compare health patterns across these three generations of my family [provide data]. What trends show improvement or worsening across generations? What factors might explain these changes?"*

Environmental and Social Context Evolution

Consider how changing environmental and social factors affect different generations:

Healthcare Access Improvements. Account for improved healthcare access and technology across generations.

Environmental Changes. Consider changes in environmental exposures as industries, regulations, and products evolved.

Lifestyle Evolution. Document different lifestyle patterns across generations, including diet, activity, and stress.

Economic and Social Context. Note economic and social factors affecting health choices in each generational cohort.

Identifying Health Patterns That Doctors Dismiss as "Genetic" Without Investigation

Challenging Medical Assumptions About Hereditary Conditions

When "Genetic" Explanations Mask Environmental Causes

Healthcare providers often attribute family health patterns to genetics without investigating environmental or lifestyle factors that might be the actual cause. Common examples include:

Autoimmune Attribution. Multiple family members with autoimmune conditions are often attributed to "genetic predisposition" without investigating shared environmental triggers.
Cancer Cluster Attribution. Cancer clusters are explained as "genetic risk" without examining occupational or environmental exposures that may actually be responsible.
Mental Health Attribution. Mental health patterns are dismissed as "hereditary" without considering trauma, socioeconomic factors, or environmental influences.

Questions to Challenge Genetic Assumptions

When healthcare providers attribute family patterns to genetics, ask specific questions:

Specific Genetic Factors. "What specific genetic factors have been identified for this condition in families like mine?"
Environmental Rule-Out. "Have environmental factors been ruled out as contributors to this family pattern?"

Genetic Testing Availability. "What genetic testing is available to confirm this hereditary risk?"
Risk Modification Options. "Are there environmental or lifestyle interventions that could modify this genetic risk?"

Researching Alternative Explanations

Environmental and Lifestyle Investigation

Use AI to research alternative explanations for family health patterns:

> *Alternative Explanation Prompt: "This condition appears in multiple family members and has been attributed to genetics. Research environmental, occupational, lifestyle, or other non-genetic factors that could explain this family pattern: [describe condition and family context]."*

Epigenetic Factors

Research how environmental factors can influence gene expression across generations:

Gene Expression Alteration. Environmental exposures can alter gene expression in ways that affect current and future generations.
Stress and Trauma Transmission. Stress and trauma effects can be passed down through epigenetic mechanisms across generations.
Nutritional Epigenetics. Nutritional factors influence genetic expression and can shape health outcomes in descendants.
Lifestyle Risk Modification. Lifestyle interventions can modify genetic risk, demonstrating that hereditary doesn't mean inevitable.

Case Study Analysis

Fibroids and Family Patterns

Consider the example of fibroids, which often "run in families" but may have significant environmental components:

Traditional Medical Approach: "Fibroids are genetic and run in your family. Surgery is the main treatment option."

Family Health Intelligence Approach:

Environmental Factor Analysis. Analyze environmental factors common to affected family members rather than defaulting to "it's genetic."
Hormonal Disruptor Research. Research hormonal disrupting chemicals that might affect multiple generations through shared exposures.
Dietary Pattern Investigation. Investigate dietary patterns that might influence fibroid development or progression.
Stress and Hormonal Health. Examine stress patterns and their relationship to hormonal health across the family.
Effective Lifestyle Interventions. Research lifestyle interventions that have shown effectiveness for reducing fibroid risk or symptoms.

> *Fibroid Family Analysis Prompt: "Research environmental and lifestyle factors that could contribute to fibroids appearing across multiple generations of a family. What non-genetic factors show strong research support as fibroid risk factors or protective factors?"*

Creating Comprehensive Family Health Profiles for Better Medical Advocacy

Building Actionable Health Profiles

Individual Risk Assessment Profiles

Create detailed health profiles for yourself based on family intelligence:

Genetic Risk Categories:

High-Priority Screening. Prioritize screening based on family patterns rather than population-level recommendations alone.
Age-Appropriate Monitoring. Develop age-appropriate monitoring strategies timed to when conditions typically appear in your family.
Evidence-Supported Lifestyle Modifications. Implement lifestyle modifications with the strongest research support for your specific risks.
Exposures to Avoid. Identify environmental exposures to avoid or minimize based on family vulnerabilities.

Protective Factor Analysis:

Unaffected Family Members. Study family members who didn't develop expected conditions to learn what may have protected them.
Protective Lifestyle or Environmental Factors. Identify lifestyle or environmental factors that might be protective within your family.
Beneficial Interventions. Note interventions that showed benefit in family members who managed conditions well.
Prevention Timing. Determine timing factors for optimal prevention strategies based on family onset patterns.

Strategic Healthcare Communication

Presenting Family Health Intelligence to Providers

Transform your family health research into compelling medical communication:

Family Health Summary Format:

Pattern Overview. Create a clear summary of concerning health patterns to present to providers.
Timeline Analysis. Include ages of onset and progression patterns that help providers assess your risk timeline.
Environmental Context. Provide relevant exposures and lifestyle factors that add context to the family pattern.
Research Integration. Integrate current research on prevention and early detection to support your requests.
Specific Requests. Make specific requests for tests, referrals, or monitoring rather than leaving it open-ended.

> *Healthcare Communication Prompt: "Help me organize this family health information into a clear, professional summary for my healthcare provider: [provide data]. Focus on actionable patterns that should influence my screening, monitoring, or prevention strategies."*

Advanced Screening Advocacy

Use family health intelligence to advocate for:

Earlier Screening. Advocate for earlier screening than standard guidelines recommend when family history warrants it.
Comprehensive Testing. Request more comprehensive testing based on family patterns rather than minimum-standard screening.
Specialist Prevention Referrals. Pursue specialist referrals for prevention counseling when family risk is significant.

Genetic Counseling. Consider genetic counseling when appropriate to formally assess hereditary risk.

Alternative Screening Methods. Explore alternative screening methods that might be more effective for your risk profile.

Creating Multi-Generational Health Action Plans

Prevention Strategy Development

Develop comprehensive prevention plans based on family patterns:

High-Priority Prevention Areas:

Strong-History Conditions. Address conditions with strong family history requiring immediate attention as top priorities.

Pattern-Based Exposure Avoidance. Avoid environmental exposures to avoid based on family patterns of susceptibility.

Risk-Specific Lifestyle Modifications. Implement lifestyle modifications with strongest research support for your specific risks.

Optimized Screening Schedules. Develop screening schedules optimized for your family patterns rather than generic timelines.

Medium-Priority Monitoring:

Moderate-History Conditions. Monitor conditions with moderate family history even when they don't require immediate intervention.

Risk-Modifying Lifestyle Factors. Track lifestyle factors that might increase or decrease risk over time.

Moderate Environmental Concerns. Stay aware of environmental factors that are not immediately concerning but worth watching.

Research and Monitoring Plan:

New Research Monitoring. Identify new research to monitor related to your family patterns.
Genetic Testing Considerations. Reevaluate genetic testing considerations as technology and affordability evolve.
Family Health Updates. Track family health updates over time as new diagnoses or patterns emerge.

Using AI to Connect Family Health Dots That Traditional Medicine Misses

Advanced Pattern Recognition Strategies

Multi-Factorial Health Analysis

Use AI to identify complex relationships that human analysis might miss:

> *Complex Pattern Analysis Prompt: "Analyze this comprehensive family health data for subtle patterns that might indicate: gene-environment interactions, protective factors, timing correlations, gender-specific risks, and intervention opportunities. Look for patterns that might not be obvious from simple family history."*

Cross-Condition Pattern Recognition

Look for relationships between different health conditions in your family:

Autoimmune Clusters. Identify autoimmune conditions that cluster together within the family.
Mental-Physical Health Correlations. Examine mental health and physical health correlations that may share biological roots.

Cardiovascular-Metabolic Relationships. Track cardiovascular and metabolic condition relationships that often co-occur.
Cancer Pattern Analysis. Analyze cancer patterns that might share environmental or genetic factors across family lines.

Predictive Health Intelligence

Risk Stratification Based on Family Patterns

Use family health intelligence to better understand your personal risk levels:

High-Risk Categories:

Multiple Close Relatives Affected. Flag conditions affecting multiple close relatives as high-risk categories.
Early-Onset Conditions. Note early-onset conditions in family members, which often indicate stronger risk.
Known Genetic Components. Identify conditions with known genetic components and the testing available to confirm them.
Shared Exposures. Recognize environmental exposures shared with affected relatives as contributors to risk.

Moderate-Risk Categories:

Distant Relative Conditions. Monitor conditions affecting distant relatives as moderate-risk factors worth watching.
Late-Onset Conditions. Consider late-onset conditions in family members for aging-related planning.
Unclear Genetic Components. Track conditions with unclear genetic components that may still carry meaningful risk.
Limited Exposure Factors. Note environmental factors with limited family exposure for possible future relevance.

Research-Guided Risk Assessment: Use AI to research current understanding of genetic and environmental risk factors:

Risk Research Prompt: "Based on this family health pattern [specific details], what does current research say about my personal risk level? What prevention strategies show the strongest evidence for people with this family history?"

Longitudinal Health Planning

Life-Stage Health Strategy

Develop health strategies that account for when conditions typically appear in your family:

Young Adult Focus (20s-30s):

Early-Onset Prevention. Implement prevention strategies for conditions that appear early in your family.
Lifestyle Establishment. Establish lifestyle patterns based on family patterns while habits are still flexible.
Early Screening Considerations. Consider early screening when family history warrants deviation from standard timelines.
Reproductive Health Planning. Plan reproductive health based on family history of pregnancy and fertility patterns.

Middle Age Focus (40s-50s):

Intensified Mid-Life Screening. Intensify screening for conditions common in your family at this age.
Mid-Life Lifestyle Modifications. Make lifestyle modifications based on family patterns that become more relevant in mid-life.
Hormonal Health. Address hormonal health considerations as they shift in perimenopausal and menopausal years.

Stress Management. Adopt stress management strategies that account for mid-life stressors and family coping patterns.

Older Adult Focus (60s+):

Late-Life Monitoring. Monitor for conditions that typically appear later in your family.
Existing Condition Management. Develop management strategies for existing conditions informed by family experience.
Quality of Life Optimization. Optimize quality of life based on family experiences with similar conditions.

Advanced Family Health Intelligence Techniques

Genealogical Health Research

Using Genealogy Tools for Health Intelligence

Combine genealogical research with health analysis:

Deceased Relative Records. Gather medical records from deceased relatives when available through family or archives.
Death Certificates. Obtain death certificates with cause of death information for older generations.
Historical Health Records. Preserve historical health records and family documents that may contain health clues.
Geographic and Occupational History. Research geographic and occupational history to understand exposures and risks.

Historical Health Context Research

Research historical health patterns in your family's geographic and cultural context:

> *Historical Context Prompt: "Research common health conditions and environmental exposures for [ethnic/geographic background] populations during [time periods when family members lived]. What health patterns were common, and what might this suggest about my family's health history?"*

Precision Prevention Planning

Personalized Prevention Based on Family Intelligence

Develop prevention strategies that account for your unique family patterns:

Nutrition Optimization:

Protective Dietary Patterns. Adopt dietary patterns that seemed protective in your family.
Family Nutritional Deficiencies. Watch for nutritional deficiencies common in your family line and correct them proactively.
Family Food Sensitivities. Identify food sensitivities or allergies with family patterns so you can avoid or test for them.
Cultural Dietary Practices. Evaluate cultural dietary practices and their health impacts across generations.

Exercise and Movement Strategies:

Healthy Activity Patterns. Adopt physical activity patterns among healthy family members as models for your own.
Condition-Based Exercise Guidance. Follow exercise limitations or recommendations based on family conditions.

Longevity Movement Strategies. Emulate movement strategies that supported longevity in your family.

Stress Management and Mental Health:

Effective Family Stress Approaches. Adopt stress management approaches that worked for other family members.
Mental Health Patterns and Interventions. Study mental health patterns and effective interventions across generations.
Multigenerational Trauma Patterns. Recognize trauma patterns that might affect multiple generations through epigenetic or behavioral mechanisms.
Resilience Factors. Identify resilience factors present in thriving family members and cultivate them in your own life.

Technology-Enhanced Family Health Tracking

Digital Family Health Management

Use technology to maintain and analyze family health information:

Health Information Management Systems:

Secure Digital Storage. Use secure digital storage for family health records with encryption and backup.
Regular Updates. Maintain regular updates with new family health information as diagnoses and events occur.
Personal Health Integration. Integrate family health information with your personal health tracking for pattern analysis.
Provider Sharing. Share appropriate information with healthcare providers in a structured, digestible format.

Predictive Analysis Tools:

Ongoing Analysis. Conduct regular analysis of new family health developments as they emerge.
Research Integration. Integrate new research with family patterns to update your understanding of risk.
Updated Risk Assessments. Produce updated risk assessments based on changing information about the family.
Prevention Strategy Monitoring. Monitor the effectiveness of preventive strategies over time and adjust as needed.

Transforming Family History from Fatalism to Empowerment

Mastering family health history intelligence transforms you from someone who passively accepts "it runs in the family" to an active participant in your health destiny. By understanding the complex interplay between genetics, environment, and lifestyle that creates family health patterns, you gain the power to intervene effectively.

The comprehensive family health intelligence you've developed becomes a powerful tool for medical advocacy, prevention planning, and early intervention. Instead of waiting for conditions to develop, you can implement evidence-based prevention strategies tailored to your specific family patterns.

Remember that family history is not destiny—it's intelligence. The patterns you've identified represent opportunities for intervention, prevention, and optimization. Your family's health challenges become the foundation for your health advantages when you understand them deeply and act strategically.

Your AI-enhanced family health intelligence system now provides you with insights that most healthcare providers have never seen and most patients never develop. This intelligence becomes the foundation for all your future healthcare decisions, from screening schedules to lifestyle choices to treatment options.

In the next chapter, we'll build on this foundation to develop strategic approaches to symptom communication and medical advocacy. Your comprehensive understanding of family health patterns will inform how you present symptoms, request testing, and advocate for care that accounts for your unique risk profile and family health intelligence.

Exercise 3.1 – Your Three-Generation Map

Draw or write a simple family tree covering yourself, your parents, and your grandparents. Next to each person, list the health conditions they had and the ages when those conditions developed.

Reflection: *What patterns do you see across generations that you've never connected to your own health before?*

Exercise 3.2 – The Conversations You Need to Have

List the family members you need to talk to about health history and what specific questions you need to ask each of them. Then commit to one conversation you'll have within the next 30 days.

Reflection: *What are you afraid of learning from these conversations? What are you afraid of not knowing?*

4

STRATEGIC SYMPTOM COMMUNICATION AND MEDICAL ADVOCACY

The Art of Medical Translation

The fifteen-minute medical appointment is a battlefield where your health outcomes are determined not just by your symptoms, but by how effectively you communicate those symptoms to a healthcare provider who may be operating under time pressure, algorithmic bias, and outdated assumptions about your demographic. The difference between receiving appropriate care and being dismissed often comes down to your ability to translate your lived experience into medical language that commands attention and respect.

Most patients approach medical appointments as passive recipients of care, hoping their healthcare provider will ask the right questions and make the correct connections. This approach fails catastrophically when you're dealing with complex symptoms, conditions that present atypically in your demographic, or providers who are influenced by unconscious bias or algorithmic decision support systems.

This chapter will transform you into a strategic medical communicator who can research symptoms effectively, prepare compelling evidence-based presentations, advocate for appropriate testing and referrals, and navigate the complex dynamics of healthcare relationships to achieve better outcomes.

How to Research and Articulate Symptoms Effectively to Healthcare Providers

Moving Beyond "I Don't Feel Well"

Understanding Medical Language and Frameworks

Healthcare providers think in terms of differential diagnoses, risk stratification, and evidence-based protocols. To communicate effectively with them, you need to understand how they process information and present your symptoms in ways that align with their decision-making frameworks.

Symptom Characterization Framework

Transform vague symptom descriptions into precise medical communication:

Instead of: "I'm tired all the time" **Strategic presentation**: "I'm experiencing persistent fatigue that began six months ago, interferes with normal daily activities, isn't relieved by rest, and is accompanied by cognitive dysfunction including difficulty concentrating and word-finding problems."

Symptom Documentation Strategy

Use AI to help organize symptom information systematically:

Symptom Organization Prompt: "Help me organize these symptoms into a clear, medical presentation format: [list symptoms with timing, triggers, severity, impact]. Include relevant medical terminology and suggest questions I should ask about potential causes."

Systematic Symptom Research Approaches

Pre-Appointment Research Protocol

Phase 1: Symptom Cluster Analysis Research how your specific combination of symptoms appears in medical literature:

Symptom Research Prompt: "Research medical literature on this combination of symptoms: [list primary symptoms]. What conditions commonly present with this symptom cluster, particularly in [your demographic]? What are red flag symptoms that require immediate attention?"

Phase 2: Demographic-Specific Presentations Research how conditions present differently in your specific demographic:

Demographic Research Prompt: "How do [suspected conditions] present differently in [your age/gender/ethnicity] compared to the typical presentation described in standard medical literature? What symptoms are commonly missed or dismissed in people like me?"

Phase 3: Differential Diagnosis Research Understand the range of conditions that could explain your symptoms:

Differential Diagnosis Prompt: "What conditions should be considered in the differential diagnosis for [your symptom cluster]? What tests or assessments would help distinguish between these possibilities?"

Strategic Symptom Presentation Techniques

The SOCRATES Method for Symptom Description

Adapt this medical assessment framework for patient communication:

Site: Where exactly is the problem located? **Onset:** When did it start and how did it develop? **Character:** What does it feel like? (Use specific descriptive terms) **Radiation:** Does it spread to other areas? **Associations:** What other symptoms occur with it? **Time course:** How has it changed over time? **Exacerbating/Relieving factors:** What makes it better or worse? **Severity:** Rate impact on function, not just pain scales

Timeline Documentation Strategy

Create clear symptom timelines that healthcare providers can quickly understand:

> *Timeline Creation Prompt: "Help me create a clear medical timeline for these symptoms: [provide symptom history]. Organize it chronologically and highlight patterns, triggers, and changes that might be medically significant."*

Functional Impact Assessment

Healthcare providers need to understand how symptoms affect your life:

Lost Activities. List specific activities you can no longer perform due to your symptoms.
Cognitive Changes. Document changes in cognitive function or memory that affect daily tasks.
Work, Relationship, and Daily Impact. Describe the impact on work, relationships, and daily activities in concrete terms.
Sleep Changes. Record sleep pattern changes and the effects they have on function and recovery.

Exercise Tolerance Changes. Note changes in exercise tolerance or physical capabilities over time.

Preparing for Medical Appointments Using AI Research and Data

Comprehensive Pre-Appointment Preparation

Medical Research Portfolio Development

Create a systematic approach to appointment preparation that demonstrates your informed participation:

Research Documentation Package:

Symptom Summary. Prepare a symptom summary organized using medical frameworks that providers will recognize.
Relevant Research. Include relevant research on conditions that might explain your symptoms.
Family History Analysis. Provide family history analysis relevant to your current concerns.
Timeline Documentation. Include timeline documentation of symptom development and changes over time.
Prioritized Question List. Prepare a question list prioritized by importance and urgency to ensure key items are covered.

AI-Assisted Question Development

Use AI to develop strategic questions that encourage thorough evaluation:

> *Question Development Prompt: "Based on my symptoms [provide summary] and research findings [provide key points], help me develop strategic questions that will encourage my healthcare provider to*

consider a comprehensive evaluation. Focus on questions that demonstrate informed participation without being confrontational."

Evidence-Based Appointment Strategy

Research Integration Techniques

Citing Relevant Studies: When appropriate, reference specific research that supports your concerns:

Demographic Presentation Citation. "Recent studies show that [condition] presents differently in women, with symptoms like [your symptoms] being more common than the classic presentation."
Test Sensitivity Citation. "Research indicates that [specific test] has higher sensitivity for detecting [condition] in [your demographic]."
Symptom Combination Citation. "Studies have found that [your symptom combination] warrants evaluation for [specific conditions]."

Professional Language Usage: Use medical terminology appropriately to demonstrate knowledge while avoiding confrontational language:

Possibility Framing. "I'd like to discuss the possibility of [condition] given my symptom cluster."
Differential Exploration. "Could we explore differential diagnoses that include [specific conditions]?"
Rule-Out Framing. "What would help us rule out [condition] given my family history and current symptoms?"

Documentation and Communication Strategy

Written Communication Preparation

Prepare written documentation that supports verbal communication:

Symptom Summary Document:

One-Page Concern Summary. Prepare a one-page summary of primary concerns that providers can review quickly.
Symptom Development Timeline. Include a timeline of symptom development to show progression.
Functional Impact Assessment. Provide a functional impact assessment showing how symptoms affect daily life.
Relevant Family History. Include relevant family history that supports diagnostic consideration.
Specific Questions and Requests. List specific questions and requests to guide the appointment.
Research Summary:
Literature Review Findings. Summarize key findings from medical literature review relevant to your case.
Demographic-Relevant Studies. Include studies relevant to your demographic and symptoms.
Diagnostic and Treatment Information. Provide information about diagnostic approaches or treatments you'd like to discuss.
Research-Generated Questions. Include questions raised by your research for discussion.

> *Document Organization Prompt: "Help me organize this information into a clear, professional one-page summary for my healthcare provider: [provide all relevant information]. Focus on the most important points that will help guide our conversation productively."*

Building Evidence-Based Arguments for Diagnostic Testing and Treatment Options

Strategic Advocacy for Appropriate Testing

Understanding Test Justification Frameworks

Healthcare providers operate within systems that require justification for testing and referrals. Understanding these frameworks helps you advocate more effectively:

Clinical Indication Requirements: Tests must have clear medical justification **Cost-Effectiveness Considerations**: Providers balance test costs with diagnostic yield **Algorithm-Based Recommendations**: Many systems use algorithms to guide testing decisions **Insurance Coverage Factors**: Coverage policies influence testing recommendations

Research-Based Testing Advocacy

Use medical literature to support requests for specific testing:

> *Testing Advocacy Prompt: "Research the clinical indicators and medical guidelines for [specific test] in patients with [your symptoms/demographics]. What evidence supports this testing in someone with my presentation? How should I present this information to my healthcare provider?"*

Overcoming Testing Resistance

Common Reasons for Test Refusal and Strategic Responses

"Let's wait and see": Response: "Given my family history of [condition] and current symptoms, what specific timeline and criteria would you recommend for monitoring versus testing? What symptoms would prompt immediate evaluation?"

"You're too young for that condition": Response: "I understand this condition is more common in older patients, but research shows it does occur in younger people, particularly those with [your risk factors]. Could we discuss early detection approaches?"

"These symptoms are probably stress-related": Response: "I'd like to rule out medical causes before attributing this to stress. What tests would help us distinguish between medical and psychological causes for these symptoms?"

Alternative Testing Strategies

When initial requests are denied, research alternative approaches:

> *Alternative Testing Prompt: "If [preferred test] isn't available or recommended, what alternative tests or assessments could help evaluate [your condition/symptoms]? What less expensive or more accessible tests might provide useful information?"*

Treatment Option Research and Advocacy

Evidence-Based Treatment Exploration

Research treatment options before discussing them with providers:

> *Treatment Research Prompt: "Research current evidence-based treatment options for [condition/symptoms], focusing on treatments that have shown effectiveness in [your demographic]. Include both conventional and integrative approaches with research support."*

Personalized Treatment Planning

Advocate for treatment approaches that consider your individual circumstances:

Family Treatment Responses. Consider previous treatment responses in your family that may predict your own.
Lifestyle Factors. Factor in lifestyle considerations that might affect treatment choices and adherence.
Interaction Potential. Evaluate potential interactions with existing conditions or medications.
Personal Preferences. Incorporate your personal preferences and values regarding treatment approaches.

When and How to Seek Second Opinions Strategically

Strategic Second Opinion Planning

Determining When Second Opinions Are Warranted

Use clear criteria to decide when second opinions are medically and strategically appropriate:

Clinical Indicators for Second Opinions:

Persistent Undiagnosed Symptoms. Persistent symptoms without clear diagnosis after reasonable evaluation indicate a second opinion is warranted.
Incomplete Diagnostic Fit. Diagnoses that don't fully explain your symptom pattern suggest further evaluation is needed.
Research-Inconsistent Recommendations. Treatment recommendations that seem inconsistent with current research deserve independent review.

Major Treatment Decisions. Major treatment decisions including surgery or long-term medication always justify a second opinion.
Dismissive Encounters. Situations where you feel dismissed or not heard are valid reasons to seek a second opinion.

Research-Based Second Opinion Strategy

> *Second Opinion Research Prompt: "Based on my situation [provide summary], research the medical indications for seeking a second opinion. What are the best practices for obtaining meaningful second opinions in cases like mine?"*

Second Opinion Implementation

Choosing Appropriate Second Opinion Sources

Different Healthcare Systems: Avoid providers within the same health system who might share similar approaches or protocols

Specialized Expertise: Seek second opinions from specialists relevant to your symptoms or suspected conditions

Academic Medical Centers: Teaching hospitals often provide comprehensive evaluation approaches

Integrative Medicine Providers: Consider providers who combine conventional and evidence-based complementary approaches

Preparation for Second Opinion Consultations

Prepare differently for second opinion appointments:

Complete Medical Record Sharing: Provide all relevant medical records, test results, and imaging

Independent Symptom Summary: Present your symptoms as if meeting a provider for the first time

Specific Questions: Focus on areas where you need clarity or alternative perspectives

Open-Minded Approach: Be prepared to hear different interpretations of your symptoms or condition

Navigating Conflicting Medical Opinions

When Second Opinions Differ Significantly

Use systematic approaches to evaluate conflicting medical advice:

> *Opinion Analysis Prompt: "I've received different medical opinions about my condition: [summarize different recommendations]. Help me research the evidence base for each approach and develop questions to help me make an informed decision about which direction to pursue."*

Collaborative Approach to Conflicting Opinions

Evidence Review: Research the evidence base for different recommendations **Risk-Benefit Analysis**: Evaluate potential risks and benefits of different approaches **Timeline Considerations**: Consider whether decisions need to be made immediately or allow time for further evaluation **Third Opinion Consultation**: Sometimes a third opinion from a different type of specialist can provide clarity

Documenting Medical Interactions and Tracking Healthcare Outcomes

Systematic Documentation Strategies

Real-Time Appointment Documentation

Develop systems for capturing important information during medical appointments:

Preparation for Documentation:

Bring Notes Tools. Bring a notebook or use a phone app for notes during the appointment.
Bring a Trusted Person. Consider bringing a trusted person to help listen and remember what's discussed.
Prepare Questions in Advance. Prepare questions in advance to ensure they get answered during limited appointment time.
Request Written Summaries. Request written summaries of recommendations or diagnoses before leaving.

Post-Appointment Documentation Process:

Immediate Post-Appointment Notes. Write detailed notes immediately after appointments while information is fresh.
Document Exact Quotes. Document exact quotes when providers make concerning statements.
Record Specifics. Record specific recommendations, medications, or follow-up instructions verbatim.
Unanswered Questions. Note questions that weren't adequately answered so you can follow up.

Healthcare Outcome Tracking

Long-Term Health Pattern Documentation

Create systems to track healthcare effectiveness over time:

Treatment Response Tracking:

Treatment-Linked Symptom Changes. Track symptom changes in response to treatments to measure real effect.
Side Effects and Reactions. Document side effects or adverse reactions as they occur.
Functional Change Measures. Measure functional improvement or decline objectively where possible.
Quality of Life Impact. Conduct quality of life impact assessments for each treatment.

Provider Performance Assessment:

Diagnostic Accuracy Over Time. Evaluate accuracy of diagnoses over time by tracking which held up under further investigation.
Treatment Recommendation Effectiveness. Assess effectiveness of treatment recommendations against actual outcomes.
Communication Quality. Evaluate communication quality and respect for patient concerns across visits.
Openness to Alternatives. Rate willingness to consider alternative approaches when initial treatments fail.

> *Outcome Tracking Prompt: "Help me create a systematic approach to tracking my healthcare outcomes, including symptom changes, treatment responses, and provider effectiveness. What metrics should I monitor to evaluate whether my healthcare is improving my condition?"*

Using Documentation for Advocacy

Building Medical History Portfolios

Compile comprehensive medical history documentation that supports future advocacy:

Comprehensive Medical Timeline:

Chronological Symptom Development. Document chronological symptom development from earliest appearance onward.
All Diagnostic Tests. Include all diagnostic tests and results with normal ranges and interpretations.
Treatment Attempts and Responses. Record all treatment attempts and responses to each.
Provider Interactions. Document provider interactions and outcomes to build a complete picture.

Pattern Documentation:

Recurring Patterns. Identify recurring symptoms or health patterns across months or years.
Diagnostic Response Clues. Track treatment responses that provide diagnostic clues about underlying causes.
Family History Correlations. Map family history correlations with your health patterns.
Environmental and Lifestyle Triggers. Note environmental or lifestyle factors that affect symptoms.

Advocacy Documentation Package:

Persistent Symptom Evidence. Compile evidence of persistent symptoms despite treatment as the foundation of your advocacy case.

Dismissal Documentation. Document provider dismissal or inadequate evaluation when it occurs.
Alternative Approach Research. Include research supporting alternative diagnostic or treatment approaches.
Clear Requests. Make clear requests for specific evaluation or referral rather than vague asks.

Advanced Medical Advocacy Strategies

Systemic Advocacy Approaches

Working Within Healthcare Systems

Patient Portal Utilization: Use electronic health record patient portals strategically:

Pre-Appointment Questions. Send written questions before appointments to ensure they're addressed during limited visit time.
Request All Records. Request copies of all test results and provider notes through the portal.
Written Concern Documentation. Document concerns in writing to create permanent records that can be referenced later.
Follow-Up on Open Items. Follow up on unanswered questions or promised callbacks in writing.

Administrative Advocacy: When clinical advocacy fails, consider administrative approaches:

Patient Relations. Contact patient relations departments for communication concerns that clinical staff cannot resolve.
Medical Directors. Escalate to medical directors for clinical care quality issues requiring oversight.

Insurance Advocacy. Use insurance advocacy channels for coverage disputes affecting your care.
Professional Licensing Boards. File with professional licensing boards for serious misconduct concerns.

Collaborative Healthcare Relationships

Building Effective Provider Partnerships

Mutual Respect Frameworks: Establish relationships based on mutual expertise:

Acknowledge Provider and Patient Expertise. Acknowledge provider medical expertise while asserting your expertise about your body.
Informed Participation. Demonstrate informed participation without challenging provider competence directly.
Collaborative Problem-Solving. Focus on collaborative problem-solving rather than adversarial interactions.
Express Appreciation. Express appreciation for thorough evaluation and open communication when providers deliver it.

Long-Term Relationship Management:

Document Effective Providers. Document positive interactions and effective providers for future reference.
Bias-Aware Networks. Build networks of healthcare providers who demonstrate bias awareness.
Maintain Quality Relationships. Maintain relationships with providers who listen and respond appropriately over time.
Refer Others to Quality Providers. Refer friends and family to providers who demonstrate quality care.

Crisis Communication Strategies

Emergency Situation Advocacy

Prepare for healthcare emergencies when advocacy becomes critical:

Emergency Information Packets:

Medical Summary Cards. Carry medical summary cards with critical information for emergency responders.
Conditions and Medications List. Include a current list of conditions, medications, and allergies.
Provider Emergency Contacts. Maintain emergency contact information for your key healthcare providers.
Advance Directives. Include advance directives and healthcare proxy information in an accessible location.

Emergency Advocacy Scripts: Prepare key phrases for emergency situations:

Condition History Statement. "I have a history of [condition] that can present as [symptoms]."
Previous Treatment Statement. "My previous episodes of [condition] required [specific treatment]."
Specialist Contact Statement. "Please contact my specialist Dr. [name] who has my complete medical history."
Advocate Request Statement. "I need someone to advocate for me — please call [emergency contact]."

Technology and Communication Enhancement

Digital Communication Tools

Telemedicine and Virtual Care Optimization

Use technology strategically for healthcare communication:

Virtual Appointment Preparation:

Test Technology in Advance. Test technology in advance to avoid communication barriers during the appointment.
Prepare Screen-Share Materials. Prepare visual aids or written materials to share on screen.
Lighting and Camera Setup. Ensure good lighting and camera positioning for symptom demonstration.
Backup Communication. Have backup communication methods ready in case technology fails.

Digital Health Integration: Use health tracking apps and wearable devices to support medical communication:

Shareable Symptom Data. Maintain symptom tracking data that can be shared with providers.
Objective Health Metrics. Capture objective health metrics that support symptom reports.
Long-Term Pattern Documentation. Produce pattern documentation over time for trend analysis.
EHR Integration. Pursue integration with electronic health records when possible to streamline sharing.

AI-Enhanced Communication Support

Real-Time Communication Support

Use AI tools to enhance medical communication:

> *Communication Support Prompt: "I'm preparing for a medical appointment about [condition/symptoms]. Help me anticipate likely questions from my healthcare provider and prepare clear, concise answers that demonstrate informed participation."*

Post-Appointment Analysis and Follow-Up:

> *Follow-Up Planning Prompt: "Based on my recent medical appointment [summarize key points], help me plan appropriate follow-up actions. What questions should I ask if symptoms don't improve? When should I seek additional evaluation?"*

Mastering Medical Communication for Better Outcomes

Strategic symptom communication and medical advocacy represent fundamental skills for navigating modern healthcare systems effectively. By preparing systematically, communicating strategically, and documenting consistently, you transform from a passive patient into an informed healthcare consumer who achieves better outcomes.

The frameworks and techniques outlined in this chapter provide you with tools to bridge the communication gap between your lived experience and medical decision-making processes. When you can articulate symptoms clearly, present research appropriately, and advocate strategically, you increase the likelihood of receiving thorough evaluation and appropriate care.

Remember that effective medical communication is not about being confrontational or challenging provider expertise inappropriately. Instead, it's about becoming an informed partner in your healthcare who can contribute meaningfully to diagnostic and treatment decisions.

Your ability to research symptoms, prepare compelling presentations, and advocate strategically becomes particularly important when dealing with conditions that present atypically in your demographic or when working with providers who may be influenced by bias or algorithmic decision support systems.

In the next chapter, we'll build on these communication skills to explore AI-powered health data analysis and lab result interpretation. The combination of strategic communication and sophisticated data analysis creates a comprehensive approach to healthcare advocacy that can dramatically improve your health outcomes and medical experience.

Exercise 4.1 – Your Symptom Timeline

Pick one ongoing symptom or health concern. Write a complete timeline: when it started, how it's changed, what triggers it, what helps, what treatments you've tried, and what questions you still have.

Reflection: *How would you describe this symptom to a doctor in 60 seconds using the SBAR method (Situation, Background, Assessment, Recommendation)?*

Exercise 4.2 – Your Next Appointment Preparation

Imagine your next medical appointment. Write down the three most important questions you want answered, the specific tests you want to discuss, and the outcomes you're hoping for. Bring this page with you.

Reflection: *What will you do if the provider dismisses or rushes through your concerns?*

5

AI-POWERED HEALTH DATA ANALYSIS AND LAB RESULT INTERPRETATION

Beyond "Normal" and "Abnormal"

Your lab results arrive through your patient portal with a simple classification: "normal" or "abnormal." Your healthcare provider spends thirty seconds reviewing dozens of values, focusing only on results that fall outside the reference ranges provided by the laboratory. This approach misses crucial health information that could predict future problems, optimize current wellness, or reveal patterns that suggest underlying conditions.

The standard approach to lab result interpretation assumes that "normal" ranges apply equally to all demographics, that trending within normal ranges isn't clinically significant, and that optimal health is the same as absence of disease. These assumptions leave massive gaps in health optimization and early disease detection, particularly for women and minorities whose optimal ranges may differ significantly from population averages.

This chapter will teach you to become a sophisticated interpreter of your own health data, using AI tools to identify trends, understand optimal versus normal ranges, recognize patterns that suggest emerging health issues, and track improvements or declines that your healthcare providers might miss. You'll learn to transform routine lab work into powerful health intelligence that guides prevention strategies and optimization efforts.

Understanding Your Lab Results Beyond the Basic "Normal" Range

The Limitations of Standard Reference Ranges

How Reference Ranges Are Established

Laboratory reference ranges are typically based on the middle 95% of values from a "healthy" population, but this approach has significant limitations:

Population Bias. Reference ranges often reflect the demographics of people who get tested, not true population health.
Disease Inclusion. "Healthy" populations used to build ranges may include people with undiagnosed conditions.
Demographic Averaging. Ranges that work for 25-year-old men may not be optimal for 45-year-old women.
Static Interpretation. Reference ranges don't account for individual variation or trending patterns in your personal health.

Individual Variation and Optimal Ranges

Your optimal ranges may differ significantly from laboratory reference ranges based on:

Age-Specific Variation. Age-specific variations in hormones and metabolism can shift your optimal range.
Gender Differences. Gender differences in iron stores, hormone levels, and cardiovascular markers affect interpretation.
Ethnic Variation. Ethnic variations in genetic factors affect lab values in ways reference ranges don't capture.
Personal Baseline. Individual baseline values represent your personal optimal function and matter more than population averages.

> *Optimal Range Research Prompt: "Research optimal ranges for [specific lab values] for someone with my demographics [age/gender/ethnicity]. How do these compare to standard reference ranges, and what do current medical guidelines recommend for optimal levels?"*

Strategic Lab Result Analysis Framework

Comprehensive Lab Review System

Develop a systematic approach to analyzing your lab results that goes beyond simple normal/abnormal classification:

Trending Analysis: Look at how values change over time, even within normal ranges **Demographic Optimization**: Research optimal ranges for your specific demographic characteristics **Pattern Recognition**: Identify relationships between different lab values that might indicate emerging issues **Functional Assessment**: Understand how lab values relate to your symptoms and functional capacity

Lab Value Categorization System

Tier 1 - Critical Monitoring: Values that directly relate to your family history or current symptoms **Tier 2 - Optimization Targets**: Values that could be optimized for better health outcomes **Tier 3 - Baseline**

Tracking: Values that establish your individual baseline for future comparison

AI-Enhanced Lab Result Interpretation

Comprehensive Lab Analysis Strategy

Use AI to help interpret lab results in the context of your individual health profile:

> *Lab Analysis Prompt: "Analyze these lab results [provide specific values] for someone with my health profile: [age, gender, symptoms, family history]. What patterns or trends should I discuss with my healthcare provider? What values might benefit from optimization even if they're within normal ranges?"*

Correlation Analysis Between Lab Values

Many health insights come from understanding relationships between different lab values rather than evaluating them in isolation:

> *Correlation Analysis Prompt: "Help me understand the relationships between these lab values [provide multiple results]. What patterns might indicate metabolic dysfunction, hormonal imbalances, nutritional deficiencies, or emerging health issues?"*

Using AI to Identify Trends and Patterns in Your Health Data Over Time

Longitudinal Health Data Analysis

Trend Identification Strategies

Tracking lab values over time reveals health patterns that single results cannot provide:

Directional Trends: Values consistently moving toward or away from optimal ranges **Seasonal Patterns:** Variations that correlate with time of year or environmental factors **Intervention Responses**: How lab values change in response to lifestyle modifications or treatments **Predictive Patterns**: Trending that might predict future health issues before they become clinical

Creating Personal Health Trend Analysis

Compile your historical lab data for comprehensive trend analysis:

> *Trend Analysis Prompt: "Analyze these lab values over time [provide historical data] to identify: 1) Values consistently trending in concerning directions, 2) Seasonal or cyclical patterns, 3) Changes that correlate with lifestyle modifications or treatments, 4) Early warning signs of potential health issues."*

Pattern Recognition for Early Detection

Metabolic Health Pattern Analysis

Use AI to identify early signs of metabolic dysfunction before clinical diagnosis:

Pre-Diabetes Indicators: Trending fasting glucose, insulin resistance markers, inflammatory indicators **Cardiovascular Risk Patterns:** Lipid ratios, inflammatory markers, homocysteine levels **Thyroid Function Trends:** TSH, T3, T4 patterns that might indicate emerging dysfunction **Hormonal Pattern Analysis:** Sex hormone trends that might affect multiple body systems

> *Metabolic Pattern Prompt: "Based on these trending lab values [provide data], what early signs of metabolic dysfunction should I monitor? What patterns suggest I should request additional testing or consider preventive interventions?"*

Nutritional Deficiency Pattern Recognition

Identify nutritional deficiencies before they become symptomatic:

Micronutrient Trending: B-vitamins, vitamin D, iron studies, magnesium **Functional Markers:** Markers that indicate nutritional status even when direct measurements aren't available **Absorption Indicators:** Patterns that might suggest digestive or absorption issues **Individual Requirement Variations:** Personal factors that might increase nutritional needs

Advanced Health Data Integration

Multi-Source Health Data Analysis

Combine lab results with other health data for comprehensive analysis:

Symptom Correlation: How lab trends correlate with symptom patterns **Lifestyle Factor Integration:** How diet, exercise, sleep, and stress affect lab values **Environmental Factor Analysis:** How seasonal changes, location, or exposures affect health markers **Medication and Supplement Effects:** How interventions affect various health markers

Integrated Analysis Prompt: "Help me correlate these lab trends [provide data] with my symptom patterns [describe symptoms] and lifestyle factors [describe relevant factors]. What relationships suggest specific interventions or further investigation?"

Researching Optimal Ranges for Your Specific Demographics and Health Goals

Demographic-Specific Optimization

Age-Related Optimization Standards

Health optimization targets change throughout life stages:

Young Adult Optimization (20s-30s): Focus on establishing healthy baselines and preventing future issues **Middle Age Optimization** (40s-50s): Emphasis on metabolic health, hormone optimization, and disease prevention **Older Adult Optimization** (60s+): Balance between optimization and realistic health maintenance

Age-Specific Research Prompt: "Research optimal lab value ranges for [specific values] in [age group]. What are the targets for optimal health versus just disease prevention in this age group?"

Gender-Specific Health Optimization

Many lab values have different optimal ranges for men and women:

Hormonal Considerations: Sex hormone optimization throughout different life stages **Iron Metabolism:** Different iron needs and optimal ranges for menstruating versus post-menopausal women **Cardiovascular Markers:** Gender-specific risk factors and optimal lipid profiles **Bone Health Markers:** Gender differences in calcium metabolism and bone density optimization

Gender-Specific Research Prompt: "Research optimal ranges for [specific lab values] in [gender] aged [age range]. How do recommendations differ from general population ranges, and what factors specific to [gender] should influence target ranges?"

Personalized Health Goal Integration

Athletic Performance Optimization

If you're physically active, your optimal ranges may differ from sedentary population norms:

Exercise-Related Markers: How regular exercise affects various lab values **Performance Optimization**: Lab values that correlate with athletic performance **Recovery Indicators:** Markers that indicate adequate recovery from exercise stress **Nutrition for Athletes**: Micronutrient needs that may be higher in active individuals

Chronic Condition Management

When managing existing health conditions, optimization targets may be more specific:

Condition-Specific Targets: Optimal ranges for people with diabetes, autoimmune conditions, cardiovascular disease **Medication Interaction Considerations**: How medications affect various lab values and what adjustments might be needed **Complication Prevention**: Lab targets that help prevent progression or complications of existing conditions

Condition-Specific Research Prompt: "For someone with [specific condition], what are the optimal lab value targets for [specific markers]? How do these differ from general population recommendations, and what additional markers should be monitored?"

Identifying Potential Health Issues Before They Become Clinical Problems

Early Detection Strategies

Subclinical Dysfunction Recognition

Many health issues develop gradually, with lab abnormalities appearing before clinical symptoms:

Thyroid Dysfunction: Subtle TSH changes that might indicate emerging thyroid issues **Insulin Resistance**: Early metabolic markers that predict diabetes development **Inflammatory Processes:** Chronic low-grade inflammation that might predict various diseases **Nutrient Depletion**: Declining nutrient stores that could affect multiple body systems

> *Early Detection Analysis Prompt: "Based on these lab trends [provide data], what subclinical health issues might be developing? What additional testing could help identify emerging problems before they become symptomatic?"*

Risk Stratification Using Lab Data

Use comprehensive lab analysis to assess future health risks:

Cardiovascular Risk Assessment: Beyond basic cholesterol panels to comprehensive cardiovascular risk markers **Metabolic Risk Evaluation**: Early indicators of metabolic syndrome development **Autoimmune Risk Markers**: Inflammatory patterns that might suggest autoimmune development **Cancer Risk Indicators**: While not diagnostic, certain patterns might suggest increased surveillance needs

Preventive Intervention Planning

Lab-Guided Prevention Strategies

Use lab trends to guide preventive interventions before problems become clinical:

Nutritional Intervention Planning: Targeted supplementation based on trending deficiencies **Lifestyle Modification Targeting**: Specific exercise, diet, or stress management approaches based on lab patterns **Monitoring Schedule Optimization**: Frequency of lab monitoring based on individual risk patterns **Specialist Referral Timing**: When trending lab values suggest need for specialized evaluation

> *Prevention Planning Prompt: "Based on these lab trends and patterns [provide data], what preventive interventions show the strongest evidence for someone with my profile? What lifestyle modifications, supplements, or monitoring strategies should I consider?"*

Creating Personalized Health Monitoring Systems

Comprehensive Health Tracking Framework

Individual Health Dashboard Development

Create a systematic approach to tracking your health data over time:

Core Monitoring Panel: Essential lab values to track based on your individual risk factors **Trending Analysis System**: How to identify significant changes versus normal variation **Intervention Tracking**: How to assess whether lifestyle changes or treatments are working **Goal**

Setting Framework: How to establish realistic health optimization targets

Technology Integration for Health Monitoring

Digital Health Record Integration: Systematic storage and analysis of lab results over time **Wearable Device Data:** How to integrate activity, sleep, and physiological data with lab results **Symptom Tracking Correlation:** Connecting subjective symptoms with objective lab data **Environmental Factor Tracking:** How external factors might affect your health markers

Monitoring System Design Prompt: "Help me design a personalized health monitoring system that includes: key lab values to track based on my risk factors [provide factors], optimal testing frequency, and methods to correlate lab data with symptoms and lifestyle factors."

Predictive Health Analytics

Personal Health Risk Modeling

Use AI to help predict health risks based on your individual data patterns:

Genetic Risk Integration: How family history combines with current lab trends to predict future risks **Lifestyle Factor Modeling:** How your specific lifestyle patterns might affect future health outcomes **Intervention Effectiveness Prediction:** Which interventions are most likely to be effective based on your profile **Timeline Estimation:** When might emerging health issues become clinically significant

Risk Modeling Prompt: "Based on my health data trends [provide data], family history [provide relevant history], and lifestyle factors [provide details], what health risks should I prioritize for prevention? What interventions show the strongest evidence for my specific risk profile?"

Advanced Lab Analysis Techniques

Functional Medicine Approaches to Lab Interpretation

Optimal Function vs. Disease Absence

Functional medicine approaches focus on optimal function rather than just absence of disease:

Functional Range Analysis: Narrower ranges that indicate optimal function rather than just "not diseased" **System-Based Interpretation:** Understanding how different body systems interact through lab markers **Root Cause Investigation:** Using lab patterns to identify underlying causes of dysfunction **Personalized Protocol Development:** Creating interventions based on individual lab patterns

> *Functional Analysis Prompt: "Analyze these lab results [provide data] from a functional medicine perspective. What patterns suggest suboptimal function even if values are within normal ranges? What interventions might optimize these values?"*

Specialized Testing Considerations

When to Request Advanced Testing

Standard lab panels may miss important health information:

Comprehensive Nutrient Analysis: When basic B12 or vitamin D testing isn't sufficient **Advanced Lipid Analysis:** Particle size and number analysis beyond basic cholesterol panels **Inflammatory Marker Assessment:** Comprehensive inflammatory evaluation beyond basic CRP **Hormonal Comprehensive Analysis:** Complete hormonal assessment rather than basic screening

Advanced Testing Research Prompt: "Based on my health profile [provide relevant information] and current lab trends [provide data], what advanced testing might provide additional insights? What are the clinical indications for more comprehensive evaluation?"

Integration with Healthcare Providers

Collaborative Lab Review Strategies

Preparation for Provider Discussions: How to present your lab analysis and concerns effectively **Question Development**: Strategic questions that encourage comprehensive lab review **Trend Documentation**: How to present trending data to support your health concerns **Intervention Requests**: How to advocate for treatments or lifestyle interventions based on lab analysis

Provider Collaboration Prompt: "Help me prepare for a discussion with my healthcare provider about these lab trends and patterns [provide analysis]. What questions should I ask, and how can I present this information to encourage collaborative health optimization?"

Technology Tools for Health Data Analysis

Digital Health Platforms

Health Data Integration Systems

Lab Result Management: Digital systems for storing and analyzing lab results over time **Trend Visualization**: Tools that help identify patterns in health data **Correlation Analysis**: Platforms that help connect lab data with symptoms and lifestyle factors **Goal Tracking**: Systems for monitoring progress toward health optimization goals

AI-Powered Health Analysis Tools

While maintaining appropriate skepticism about commercial health AI, some tools can provide useful analysis:

Pattern Recognition Software: Tools that identify trends in personal health data **Risk Assessment Platforms:** AI systems that help stratify health risks based on multiple factors **Intervention Tracking**: Tools that help assess the effectiveness of health interventions **Predictive Analytics**: Platforms that help predict future health risks based on current data

> *Tool Evaluation Prompt: "Research reliable, evidence-based digital tools for personal health data analysis. What tools have good scientific backing for [specific health analysis needs], and how should I evaluate the credibility of health technology platforms?"*

Transforming Data into Health Intelligence

AI-powered health data analysis transforms routine lab work from a passive medical procedure into an active tool for health optimization and disease prevention. By understanding optimal ranges, identifying trends, and correlating data with symptoms and lifestyle factors, you gain insights that can guide targeted interventions and prevent health issues before they become clinical problems.

The systematic approach to lab result interpretation outlined in this chapter provides you with tools to extract maximum value from your health data while working collaboratively with healthcare providers. When you can identify concerning trends, research optimal ranges for your demographics, and present compelling data-driven arguments for interventions, you become an active partner in your health optimization rather than a passive recipient of medical care.

Remember that lab data interpretation should always be done in consultation with qualified healthcare providers. The goal is not to replace medical expertise but to become an informed partner who can contribute meaningfully to health optimization discussions and advocate for appropriate testing and interventions based on trending data.

Your AI-enhanced approach to health data analysis becomes particularly powerful when combined with the family health intelligence and strategic communication skills developed in previous chapters. The ability to identify patterns, research optimal approaches, and communicate effectively with providers creates a comprehensive framework for achieving better health outcomes through data-driven advocacy.

In the next chapter, we'll explore how to combat healthcare gaslighting and dismissive care, building on your data analysis skills to present compelling cases for appropriate medical attention when providers dismiss or minimize your health concerns.

Exercise 5.1 – Your Lab Results Inventory

List your most recent lab results (or pull them up in your patient portal). Write down any values that were flagged as abnormal AND any values that were within "normal" range but toward the edges.

____

____

____

____

____

____

____

____

____

____

____

____

Reflection: *Which results have you never questioned because they were labeled "normal"? What would it mean if "normal" wasn't actually optimal for you?*

Exercise 5.2 – Your AI Lab Analysis Prompt

Using the AI prompts from this chapter, write a specific prompt you'll use to analyze your most recent lab results. Include your age, sex, demographic background, and any relevant health conditions.

____

____

____

____

____

____

____

____

____

____

____

____

Reflection: *What patterns might emerge when you look at your*

6

MASTERING LAB WORK AND BLOOD ANALYSIS - BEYOND "NORMAL" RANGES

The Myth of Universal Normal Ranges

When your lab results arrive through your patient portal with values neatly categorized as "normal" or "abnormal," you're seeing the end result of a deeply flawed system that treats all patients as identical and equates "normal" with "optimal." This binary approach to lab interpretation misses crucial health information that could predict future problems, optimize current wellness, or reveal patterns suggesting underlying conditions that won't show up as "abnormal" until significant disease progression has occurred. The standard medical approach to laboratory results operates on outdated assumptions that reference ranges apply equally across all demographics, that values within normal ranges don't require attention, and that optimal health can be determined by comparing your results to population averages that may include significant numbers of unhealthy individuals. These assumptions create massive blind spots in health optimization and disease prevention, particularly for women and minorities whose optimal ranges often differ significantly from population-based reference standards.

Most healthcare providers spend less than sixty seconds reviewing dozens of lab values, focusing only on results that fall outside reference ranges and missing trends, patterns, and optimization opportunities that could transform your health outcomes. This assembly-line approach to lab interpretation treats your blood work as a series of isolated data points rather than an integrated picture of your body's functional status, metabolic health, and disease risk trajectory. Understanding laboratory medicine beyond the basic "normal" and "abnormal" classifications transforms routine blood work from a passive medical procedure into an active tool for health optimization, early disease detection, and personalized prevention strategies. This chapter will teach you to interpret your lab results with the sophistication of a functional medicine practitioner, identify trends and patterns that predict future health issues, understand optimal ranges for your specific demographics, and advocate effectively for comprehensive testing that reveals your complete metabolic picture.

The knowledge you'll gain provides the foundation for meaningful conversations with healthcare providers about optimization rather than just disease absence, early intervention strategies based on trending data, and personalized health approaches that account for your individual physiology rather than population averages. When you understand what your lab results actually mean, you transform from a passive recipient of medical opinions into an informed participant in health optimization.

Understanding Reference Ranges and Their Critical Limitations

The Flawed Foundation of Laboratory Medicine

How Reference Ranges Are Actually Established

The "normal" ranges printed on your lab results represent statistical averages rather than optimal health markers, and understanding this distinction is crucial for effective health advocacy. Laboratory reference ranges are typically established by testing presumably healthy populations and using the middle 95% of values as the "normal" range. This approach has fundamental problems that directly affect your health care.

Reference populations often include people with undiagnosed conditions, subclinical disease, and suboptimal health status. When laboratories establish normal ranges for cholesterol, blood sugar, or thyroid function, they include data from people who may have early-stage diabetes, cardiovascular disease, or thyroid dysfunction that hasn't been diagnosed yet. This means "normal" ranges can include values that actually indicate emerging health problems.

The 95% statistical range approach means that 5% of healthy people will always fall outside "normal" ranges, leading to unnecessary concern about values that may be perfectly healthy for individuals. Conversely, values within the normal range may indicate significant health problems for people whose optimal values fall at different points within that range.

Demographic factors significantly affect optimal lab values, but most reference ranges don't account for age, gender, ethnicity, or body composition differences. A 25-year-old athletic woman's optimal iron levels differ dramatically from those of a 65-year-old sedentary man, yet they're often compared to the same reference ranges. This one-size-fits-all approach particularly disadvantages women and minorities whose optimal values may differ from population averages.

> *Reference Range Research Prompt: "Research how laboratory reference ranges are established for [specific lab test] and what factors affect optimal values for someone with my demographics [age, gender, ethnicity, health status]. How do optimal ranges differ from standard reference ranges?"*

The Problem with Population-Based Averages

Population-based reference ranges reflect the health status of people who get laboratory testing, not necessarily healthy populations. People who need blood work often have health concerns, chronic conditions, or risk factors that skew reference ranges toward less optimal values. Additionally, geographic and socioeconomic factors affect reference populations, meaning ranges established in one location may not apply to diverse populations.

Historical bias in medical research means reference ranges often reflect predominantly male, white, middle-aged populations. Women, minorities, children, and elderly individuals may have optimal ranges that differ significantly from established reference standards. This bias particularly affects conditions that present differently across demographics or respond differently to treatment in various populations.

Seasonal and environmental factors affect many lab values, but reference ranges typically don't account for these variations. Vitamin D levels naturally fluctuate with sun exposure, inflammatory markers can vary with stress and sleep patterns, and hormone levels change throughout menstrual cycles. Static reference ranges miss these important variations that affect interpretation.

Individual Variation and Optimal Health Ranges

Understanding Your Personal Baseline

Your optimal lab values may differ significantly from population-based reference ranges based on genetic factors, lifestyle patterns, and individual physiology. Establishing your personal baseline values provides much more meaningful information than comparing single results to population averages.

Some people naturally have higher or lower values for specific markers while maintaining excellent health. Identifying your personal patterns requires tracking values over time and correlating them with symptoms, energy levels, and overall health status. This individual approach to lab interpretation provides insights that population-based ranges miss entirely.

Athletic individuals often have lab values that differ from sedentary populations. Regular exercise affects markers like creatine kinase, lactate dehydrogenase, and even some liver enzymes. Understanding exercise-related changes prevents misinterpretation of values that are actually indicators of good health and fitness.

Women's lab values fluctuate throughout menstrual cycles, pregnancy, and hormonal transitions like perimenopause and menopause. Standard reference ranges often don't account for these normal physiological changes, leading to inappropriate concern about values that are actually normal for specific life stages.

> *Personal Baseline Analysis Prompt: "Analyze my lab value trends over time [provide historical data] to identify my personal baseline patterns. What values consistently fall at specific points within reference ranges, and how do they correlate with my symptoms and health status?"*

Age-Related Optimal Range Modifications

Optimal lab values change throughout life stages, but standard reference ranges often don't reflect these changes adequately. Understanding age-appropriate optimization targets helps identify when values indicate health concerns versus normal aging processes.

Young adults typically benefit from tighter optimal ranges that support peak performance and long-term health. Values that indicate increased risk for future problems deserve attention even when they fall within normal ranges. Early intervention during this life stage provides maximum benefit for long-term health outcomes.

Middle-aged individuals face increasing disease risk, making optimal ranges more important for prevention. Metabolic markers like glucose, insulin, and lipids require closer monitoring, with optimization targets that prevent progression to clinical disease. Hormone optimization becomes increasingly important during this stage, particularly for women approaching menopause.

Older adults may have different risk-benefit considerations that affect optimal ranges. Extremely tight control of some markers may not provide benefit and could increase treatment risks. However, maintaining function and preventing frailty requires attention to markers like protein levels, vitamin status, and inflammatory indicators.

Essential Laboratory Tests Decoded: What They Really Tell You

Complete Blood Count (CBC): Your Cellular Health Foundation

Red Blood Cell Analysis Beyond Anemia Diagnosis

The complete blood count provides detailed information about your cellular health that extends far beyond simple anemia diagnosis. Understanding each component reveals insights about oxygen delivery, nutritional status, and overall physiological function.

Red blood cell count, hemoglobin, and hematocrit work together to indicate oxygen-carrying capacity. However, optimal values depend on altitude, fitness level, and individual physiology. Athletes often have higher red blood cell counts due to training adaptations, while people living at high altitudes naturally develop increased red blood cell production.

Mean corpuscular volume (MCV) indicates red blood cell size, providing clues about nutritional status and bone marrow function. Large red blood cells (high MCV) can indicate B12 or folate deficiency, even when these vitamins fall within normal ranges on direct testing. Small red blood cells (low MCV) may suggest iron deficiency or genetic conditions affecting hemoglobin production.

Red cell distribution width (RDW) measures variation in red blood cell size and provides early indicators of nutritional deficiencies, inflammation, or bone marrow problems. Increasing RDW over time can predict developing health issues before other markers become abnormal.

CBC Analysis Prompt: "Analyze my CBC results [provide specific values] for optimization opportunities beyond basic anemia screening. What do the patterns in my red blood cell indices suggest about nutritional status, oxygen delivery, and cellular health?"

White Blood Cell Patterns and Immune Function

White blood cell count and differential provide insights into immune system function, infection risk, and inflammatory status. Total white blood cell count varies significantly among healthy individuals, making personal trending more important than single values.

Neutrophil counts indicate bacterial infection risk and bone marrow function. Chronic stress, intense exercise, and certain medications can affect neutrophil levels. Understanding your baseline helps distinguish between normal variation and concerning changes.

Lymphocyte counts reflect viral immunity and overall immune system health. Low lymphocyte counts can indicate immune suppression from stress, poor nutrition, or underlying conditions. High lymphocyte counts may suggest viral infections or certain autoimmune conditions.

Eosinophil levels often indicate allergic responses or parasitic infections. Elevated eosinophils can provide early clues about food allergies, environmental sensitivities, or travel-related exposures that require investigation.

Platelet Function and Bleeding Risk Assessment

Platelet count and function affect bleeding and clotting risk. Normal platelet counts range widely, but individual patterns provide more meaningful information than single values. Trending platelet counts can identify developing problems before they become clinically significant.

Mean platelet volume (MPV) indicates platelet size and activation status. Large platelets are typically younger and more active, while small platelets may indicate bone marrow problems or certain medications effects. MPV trends provide insights into platelet production and turnover.

Comprehensive Metabolic Panel (CMP): Your Biochemical Foundation

Glucose and Metabolic Health Assessment

Fasting glucose provides crucial information about metabolic health, but interpretation requires understanding optimal ranges rather than just normal versus abnormal classifications. Current medical guidelines define normal fasting glucose as less than 100 mg/dL, but optimal metabolic health typically requires tighter ranges.

Optimal fasting glucose for metabolic health falls between 70-85 mg/dL for most people. Values above 90 mg/dL, while technically normal, indicate increased risk for developing insulin resistance and type 2 diabetes. Early intervention at this stage can prevent progression to clinical disease.

Fasting glucose variability provides important information about metabolic stability. Consistent values indicate good metabolic control, while significant fluctuations may suggest insulin resistance, stress effects, or dietary factors affecting glucose regulation.

Post-meal glucose responses, when available, provide additional insights into metabolic health. Normal individuals typically see glucose return to baseline within two hours of eating. Prolonged elevation may indicate early insulin resistance or pancreatic dysfunction.

Glucose Optimization Prompt: "Analyze my fasting glucose trends [provide historical values] and current reading [current value]. What does this pattern suggest about my metabolic health, and what optimization strategies might improve glucose regulation?"

Kidney Function Markers and Optimization

Creatinine and blood urea nitrogen (BUN) assess kidney function, but interpretation requires understanding individual factors that affect these markers. Muscle mass, age, gender, and protein intake significantly influence creatinine levels.

Estimated glomerular filtration rate (eGFR) provides age and gender-adjusted kidney function assessment. However, the equations used may not be accurate for all ethnicities, body compositions, or clinical situations. Understanding these limitations prevents misinterpretation.

BUN-to-creatinine ratio provides insights into kidney function and hydration status. High ratios may indicate dehydration, high protein intake, or kidney problems, while low ratios might suggest low protein intake or liver problems.

Cystatin C, when available, provides kidney function assessment that's less affected by muscle mass than creatinine. This alternative marker can identify kidney problems earlier or provide more accurate assessment in people with unusual body composition.

Liver Function and Metabolic Assessment

Liver enzymes (ALT, AST, alkaline phosphatase) assess liver health, but normal ranges don't necessarily indicate optimal liver function. Understanding factors that affect liver enzymes helps distinguish between concerning findings and normal variations.

ALT (alanine aminotransferase) specifically indicates liver cell damage and provides the most direct assessment of liver health. Values above 25-30 U/L may indicate liver stress even when they fall within normal ranges. Trending ALT values provides early warning of developing liver problems.

AST (aspartate aminotransferase) comes from liver, heart, and muscle tissue. Elevated AST without elevated ALT may indicate heart or muscle problems rather than liver disease. Exercise, muscle injury, and certain supplements can affect AST levels.

Alkaline phosphatase comes from the liver, bone, and intestine. Elevated levels may indicate liver problems, bone disease, or intestinal issues. Age, gender, and growth status affect normal alkaline phosphatase levels.

Protein and Nutritional Status Assessment

Total protein and albumin provide insights into nutritional status, liver function, and protein metabolism. Low protein levels may indicate poor nutrition, liver problems, kidney disease, or chronic inflammation.

Albumin specifically reflects protein synthesis by the liver and nutritional status over the previous 2-3 weeks. Low albumin can indicate poor nutrition, liver disease, kidney disease, or chronic inflammation. Optimal albumin levels support proper fluid balance and nutrient transport.

Globulin levels (calculated as total protein minus albumin) reflect immune system protein production and can indicate infections, autoimmune conditions, or liver problems. The albumin-to-globulin ratio provides additional insights into protein metabolism balance.

Advanced Lipid Analysis: Beyond Basic Cholesterol

Understanding Cholesterol Complexity

Traditional lipid panels measure total cholesterol, LDL, HDL, and triglycerides, but these basic measurements miss important information about cardiovascular risk and optimization opportunities. Advanced lipid analysis provides insights that basic panels cannot reveal.

Total cholesterol provides limited information about cardiovascular risk. Some people with high total cholesterol have low cardiovascular risk due to high HDL levels, while others with normal total cholesterol may have high risk due to small, dense LDL particles or other risk factors.

LDL cholesterol calculation (using the Friedewald equation) becomes inaccurate when triglycerides exceed 400 mg/dL. Direct LDL measurement provides more accurate results, particularly for people with high triglycerides or unusual lipid patterns.

HDL cholesterol levels vary significantly by gender, with women typically having higher levels than men. Optimal HDL levels support cardiovascular health, but extremely high levels (above 80-90 mg/dL) may sometimes indicate other health issues requiring investigation.

> *Lipid Optimization Prompt: "Analyze my lipid panel results [provide values] for cardiovascular risk optimization beyond basic guidelines. What patterns suggest metabolic dysfunction, and what interventions might improve my lipid profile?"*

Triglycerides and Metabolic Health

Triglyceride levels provide crucial information about metabolic health and insulin sensitivity. Elevated triglycerides often indicate insulin resistance, even when glucose levels remain normal. This makes triglycerides an early warning system for metabolic dysfunction.

Optimal triglyceride levels fall below 100 mg/dL for most people, with levels below 75 mg/dL indicating excellent metabolic health. Values above 150 mg/dL, while technically normal according to standard guidelines, suggest increased cardiovascular and diabetes risk.

The triglyceride-to-HDL ratio provides insights into insulin sensitivity and cardiovascular risk. Ratios above 3:1 suggest insulin resistance, while ratios below 2:1 indicate good metabolic health. This ratio often predicts diabetes risk better than glucose levels alone.

Postprandial (after-meal) triglycerides, when measured, provide additional insights into fat metabolism and cardiovascular risk. Normal individuals typically see triglycerides return to baseline within 6-8 hours of eating. Prolonged elevation indicates poor fat clearance and increased cardiovascular risk.

Advanced Lipid Markers for Precision Assessment

LDL particle number (LDL-P) and size provide more accurate cardiovascular risk assessment than basic LDL cholesterol levels. Small, dense LDL particles are more atherogenic than large, fluffy particles, even at similar cholesterol concentrations.

Apolipoprotein B (ApoB) measures the number of atherogenic particles and often provides better risk assessment than LDL cholesterol levels. Each atherogenic particle contains one ApoB molecule, making this measurement more precise than calculated LDL.

Lipoprotein(a) [Lp(a)] represents genetic cardiovascular risk that doesn't respond to typical interventions. Elevated Lp(a) requires specific treatment approaches and more aggressive management of other cardiovascular risk factors.

Metabolic Health Markers: Decoding the Diabetes Spectrum

Understanding the Glucose-Insulin Relationship

Normal Glucose Regulation Physiology

Healthy glucose regulation involves complex interactions between insulin production, tissue sensitivity, and glucose uptake. Understanding this physiology helps interpret lab values and identify optimization opportunities before clinical problems develop.

After eating, blood glucose rises, triggering insulin release from pancreatic beta cells. Insulin facilitates glucose uptake by muscle and fat cells while suppressing glucose production by the liver. In healthy individuals, this system maintains glucose levels within narrow ranges.

Insulin sensitivity determines how effectively tissues respond to insulin signals. High insulin sensitivity means small amounts of insulin effectively regulate glucose, while insulin resistance requires progressively higher insulin levels to maintain normal glucose.

Beta cell function refers to the pancreas's ability to produce adequate insulin in response to glucose levels. Early diabetes development involves both insulin resistance and declining beta cell function, though the relative contribution varies among individuals.

> *Glucose Regulation Assessment Prompt: "Based on my fasting glucose [value], HbA1c [value], and any available insulin data [value if available], assess my glucose regulation status. What does this pattern suggest about insulin sensitivity and beta cell function?"*

The Prediabetes Spectrum: Earlier Than You Think

Redefining Normal Glucose Levels

Current medical guidelines define normal fasting glucose as less than 100 mg/dL and normal HbA1c as less than 5.7%, but these thresholds miss early metabolic dysfunction that predicts future diabetes and cardiovascular problems.

Research shows increased diabetes and cardiovascular risk begins at fasting glucose levels above 85-90 mg/dL, well within the "normal" range. People with fasting glucose between 90-99 mg/dL have significantly higher diabetes risk than those with levels below 85 mg/dL.

HbA1c levels between 5.5-5.6%, while technically normal, indicate increased diabetes risk and may benefit from preventive interventions. Optimal HbA1c levels for long-term health typically fall between 4.8-5.3%.

Postprandial glucose levels provide additional insights into early metabolic dysfunction. Normal individuals typically see glucose peaks below 140 mg/dL one hour after eating and return to baseline within two hours. Higher peaks or delayed return suggest early insulin resistance.

Borderline Prediabetes: The Hidden Zone

The zone between optimal glucose levels and official prediabetes diagnosis represents a critical intervention period where lifestyle modifications can prevent progression to clinical disease. This "borderline prediabetic" zone deserves attention despite falling within normal ranges.

Fasting glucose levels between 90-99 mg/dL indicate intermediate diabetes risk. While not technically prediabetic, this range suggests insulin resistance development and benefits from preventive interventions including dietary modifications, exercise programs, and metabolic monitoring.

HbA1c levels between 5.4-5.6% similarly indicate intermediate risk. These values suggest glucose elevation over the previous 2-3 months, even when individual glucose measurements appear normal. Trending HbA1c values provides early warning of metabolic deterioration.

The concept of "metabolically healthy obesity" versus "metabolically unhealthy normal weight" illustrates that body weight alone doesn't predict metabolic dysfunction. Some normal-weight individuals develop insulin resistance and diabetes risk, while some overweight individuals maintain excellent metabolic health.

> *Borderline Risk Assessment Prompt: "Analyze my glucose-related markers [fasting glucose, HbA1c, any available insulin or c-peptide data] for early signs of metabolic dysfunction. What interventions might prevent progression to clinical prediabetes or diabetes?"*

Insulin Resistance: The Hidden Epidemic

Understanding Insulin Resistance Development

Insulin resistance develops gradually over years or decades, often beginning with normal glucose levels but elevated insulin requirements. Standard medical testing often misses early insulin resistance because glucose levels remain normal due to compensatory insulin elevation.

Fasting insulin levels provide direct assessment of insulin resistance, though this test isn't routinely ordered. Optimal fasting insulin levels typically fall below 10 mIU/L, with levels above 15 mIU/L suggesting insulin resistance even with normal glucose.

The HOMA-IR (Homeostatic Model Assessment of Insulin Resistance) calculation uses fasting glucose and insulin to estimate insulin resistance.

HOMA-IR values above 2.5 suggest insulin resistance, while values below 1.0 indicate excellent insulin sensitivity.

Insulin resistance affects multiple body systems beyond glucose regulation, including fat metabolism, inflammation, blood pressure regulation, and hormone production. This explains why insulin resistance increases risk for cardiovascular disease, PCOS, fatty liver, and other conditions.

Clinical Manifestations of Insulin Resistance

Insulin resistance often manifests through non-glucose markers that may be overlooked during routine evaluation. Recognizing these patterns helps identify insulin resistance before glucose abnormalities develop.

Triglyceride elevation often represents the earliest laboratory sign of insulin resistance. High insulin levels promote fat synthesis and storage while impairing fat breakdown, leading to elevated triglycerides even with normal glucose levels.

Low HDL cholesterol frequently accompanies insulin resistance due to altered lipid metabolism. The combination of high triglycerides and low HDL creates an atherogenic lipid pattern that increases cardiovascular risk independent of LDL levels.

Elevated blood pressure may result from insulin resistance through multiple mechanisms including sodium retention, vascular dysfunction, and sympathetic nervous system activation. Many people with "essential hypertension" actually have underlying insulin resistance.

Reversibility and Intervention Strategies

Early-stage insulin resistance often responds dramatically to lifestyle interventions, making early detection and intervention crucial for preventing progression to irreversible diabetes. Understanding reversibility potential guides treatment intensity and monitoring strategies.

Dietary interventions targeting carbohydrate intake, meal timing, and food quality can significantly improve insulin sensitivity. Low-carbohydrate diets, intermittent fasting, and elimination of processed foods often produce rapid improvements in insulin resistance markers.

Exercise interventions, particularly resistance training and high-intensity interval training, improve insulin sensitivity through multiple mechanisms including increased glucose uptake by muscle tissue and improved mitochondrial function.

Stress management and sleep optimization affect insulin sensitivity through cortisol regulation and cellular repair processes. Chronic stress and poor sleep quality can maintain or worsen insulin resistance despite excellent diet and exercise habits.

> *Insulin Resistance Reversal Strategy Prompt: "Based on my current metabolic markers [provide available data], design a comprehensive insulin resistance reversal plan. What lifestyle interventions show strongest evidence for improving insulin sensitivity in someone with my health profile?"*

Advanced Metabolic Testing and Interpretation

Continuous Glucose Monitoring Insights

Continuous glucose monitoring (CGM) provides detailed information about glucose patterns that traditional testing misses. Even people without diabetes can benefit from CGM data to optimize metabolic health and identify early dysfunction.

CGM reveals glucose variability patterns that predict metabolic health better than average glucose levels. High variability indicates metabolic instability even when average glucose remains normal. Reduced variability often results from improved diet quality and metabolic health.

Dawn phenomenon patterns show early morning glucose elevation due to hormone changes. Excessive dawn phenomenon may indicate insulin resistance or inadequate overnight glucose control. Understanding individual patterns helps optimize evening meal timing and composition.

Postprandial glucose response patterns reveal food sensitivity and metabolic function. Identifying foods that cause excessive glucose elevation allows for personalized dietary modifications that improve metabolic health.

Metabolic Flexibility Assessment

Metabolic flexibility refers to the ability to switch efficiently between glucose and fat utilization based on availability and demands. Poor metabolic flexibility contributes to insulin resistance and metabolic dysfunction.

Respiratory quotient measurements (when available) provide direct assessment of metabolic flexibility by measuring the ratio of carbon dioxide production to oxygen consumption. Values closer to 0.7 indicate fat utilization, while values near 1.0 indicate glucose utilization.

Ketone measurements, either through blood testing or urine strips, indicate fat metabolism activation. The ability to produce ketones during fasting periods or carbohydrate restriction suggests good metabolic flexibility.

Heart rate variability patterns may reflect metabolic flexibility through autonomic nervous system function. Better metabolic flexibility often correlates with improved heart rate variability and stress adaptation.

AI-Enhanced Laboratory Analysis Framework

Systematic Approach to Lab Result Interpretation

Comprehensive Data Integration Strategy

Modern lab result interpretation benefits from systematic analysis that considers multiple markers simultaneously rather than evaluating individual values in isolation. AI tools can help identify patterns and relationships that human analysis might miss.

Pattern recognition across multiple lab results often reveals insights that individual value interpretation cannot provide. Subtle changes in several related markers may indicate emerging health issues before any single value becomes abnormal.

Temporal analysis comparing current results to historical values provides more meaningful information than single-point assessment. Trending patterns reveal trajectory toward or away from optimal health, even when all values remain within normal ranges.

Demographic contextualization adjusts interpretation based on age, gender, ethnicity, and lifestyle factors that affect optimal ranges. What appears abnormal for population averages may be optimal for specific individuals, and vice versa.

> *Comprehensive Lab Analysis Prompt: "Analyze these complete lab results [provide all available values with dates] for patterns, trends, and optimization opportunities. Consider my demographics [age, gender, relevant factors] and health goals [describe goals]. What relationships between different markers suggest specific interventions?"*

Advanced Pattern Recognition Techniques

Multi-System Integration Analysis

Laboratory values reflect the integrated function of multiple body systems, and understanding these relationships provides insights that single-system analysis cannot reveal. AI analysis can identify complex patterns across different organ systems.

Metabolic-cardiovascular integration examines relationships between glucose metabolism, lipid patterns, and cardiovascular risk markers. Insulin resistance affects multiple systems simultaneously, creating recognizable patterns across seemingly unrelated tests.

Inflammatory-immune system patterns connect markers like CRP, ESR, white blood cell differential, and autoimmune markers. Chronic low-grade inflammation affects multiple body systems and may be detectable through pattern analysis before individual markers become obviously abnormal.

Nutritional-metabolic integration analyzes relationships between nutritional markers (vitamins, minerals, proteins) and metabolic function markers. Nutritional deficiencies often affect multiple systems simultaneously, creating detectable patterns in comprehensive lab panels.

Predictive Health Modeling

AI analysis can help predict future health risks based on current lab value patterns and trends. This predictive approach enables earlier interventions than waiting for clinical symptoms or obvious abnormalities.

Risk trajectory analysis examines how current lab patterns predict future disease development. Subtle changes in multiple markers may indicate increased risk for diabetes, cardiovascular disease, or other conditions before clinical diagnosis becomes possible.

Intervention effectiveness prediction uses historical response patterns to predict how specific interventions might affect lab values. This personalized approach optimizes intervention selection and monitoring strategies.

Optimization potential assessment identifies which lab values have the greatest potential for improvement and would provide the most significant health benefits if optimized. This prioritization guides intervention efforts for maximum impact.

> *Predictive Analysis Prompt: "Based on my lab value trends [provide historical data] and current results [provide current values], what future health risks should I monitor? What interventions show strongest evidence for optimizing my specific pattern of lab results?"*

Technology-Enhanced Monitoring Systems

Digital Health Integration

Modern health monitoring benefits from integration between laboratory testing and digital health tools including wearable devices, smartphone apps, and home monitoring systems. This integration provides more comprehensive health pictures than isolated lab testing.

Wearable device data correlation with lab results can reveal relationships between subjective symptoms, physiological patterns, and objective laboratory markers. Heart rate variability, sleep patterns, and activity levels often correlate with metabolic and inflammatory markers.

Symptom tracking integration connects subjective experiences with objective lab data. Understanding how lab value changes correlate with energy levels, mood, cognitive function, and physical symptoms provides personalized insights for optimization.

Environmental factor correlation examines how external factors like weather, stress levels, travel, and seasonal changes affect lab values. This understanding helps distinguish between pathological changes and normal variations.

Automated Monitoring and Alert Systems

Technology can enhance lab monitoring through automated trend analysis and alert systems that identify concerning changes before they become clinically significant. These systems provide early warning capabilities for health optimization.

Trend alert systems monitor lab value changes over time and identify concerning patterns that warrant attention. Gradual changes that remain within normal ranges might still indicate important health trends requiring intervention.

Optimization opportunity identification uses AI analysis to identify lab values with significant improvement potential and evidence-based interventions likely to be effective. This proactive approach focuses efforts on areas with greatest potential benefit.

Personalized monitoring schedule optimization adjusts testing frequency based on individual risk factors, current health status, and optimization goals. Higher-risk individuals or those implementing interventions may benefit from more frequent monitoring.

Building Comprehensive Health Monitoring Systems

Strategic Laboratory Testing Approach

Individualized Testing Protocols

Effective health monitoring requires systematic approaches to laboratory testing that account for individual risk factors, health goals, and optimization strategies. Generic testing protocols miss opportunities for personalized health management.

Baseline comprehensive assessment establishes individual normal ranges and identifies current health status across multiple systems. This comprehensive approach provides the foundation for all future monitoring and optimization efforts.

Risk-stratified monitoring adjusts testing frequency and scope based on family history, current health status, lifestyle factors, and intervention responses. Higher-risk individuals benefit from more frequent monitoring, while stable individuals may require less intensive surveillance.

Goal-oriented testing focuses on markers most relevant to individual health goals and optimization efforts. People focused on metabolic health might emphasize glucose, insulin, and lipid monitoring, while those concerned about inflammation might prioritize inflammatory markers and nutritional status.

> *Personalized Testing Strategy Prompt: "Design an optimal laboratory monitoring strategy based on my health profile [age, gender, family history, current conditions], health goals [describe goals], and risk factors [describe factors]. What tests should I prioritize, and what frequency provides an optimal cost-benefit ratio?"*

Quality Control and Result Validation

Laboratory Quality Assessment

Not all laboratory testing provides equally accurate or reliable results. Understanding laboratory quality factors helps ensure that your health decisions are based on accurate data rather than flawed testing.

Laboratory accreditation and certification indicate adherence to quality standards for testing procedures, personnel training, and quality control measures. Accredited laboratories typically provide more reliable results than non-accredited facilities.

Reference laboratory versus local laboratory trade-offs involve considerations of quality, consistency, and result interpretation. Major reference laboratories often provide more sophisticated testing and better quality control, while local laboratories may offer convenience and faster results.

Test-specific quality considerations recognize that some tests require specialized expertise or equipment that may not be available at all laboratories. Complex tests like advanced lipid analysis or specialized hormone testing may require specific laboratory capabilities.

Result Consistency and Tracking

Consistent laboratory testing improves the reliability of trend analysis and optimization monitoring. Using the same laboratory for serial testing reduces variability due to different testing methods or equipment.

Timing consistency affects many lab values, particularly hormones, glucose, and lipids. Consistent timing for blood draws improves the reliability of trend analysis and reduces variability due to circadian rhythms and meal effects.

Preparation standardization including fasting requirements, medication timing, and activity restrictions ensures consistent testing conditions. Inconsistent preparation can create artificial variability that masks real health trends.

Integration with Healthcare Provider Communication

Provider Education and Collaboration

Many healthcare providers receive limited training in optimization-focused lab interpretation beyond pathology identification. Educating providers about your health goals and optimization approach can improve collaboration and care quality.

Optimization versus pathology focus requires communication about your interest in health optimization rather than just disease detection. Providers trained in pathology-focused medicine may need education about optimization benefits and approaches.

Research presentation skills help communicate evidence-based optimization approaches to providers who may not be familiar with functional medicine or optimization strategies. Professional presentation of research improves provider receptiveness to optimization-focused care.

Collaborative goal setting ensures that provider recommendations align with your health optimization goals. Clear communication about objectives helps providers understand your priorities and adjust recommendations accordingly.

> *Provider Communication Strategy Prompt: "Help me prepare for a discussion with my healthcare provider about optimization-focused lab interpretation. What key points should I communicate about my health goals, and how can I present evidence-based optimization approaches professionally?"*

Long-Term Health Optimization Through Lab Intelligence

Predictive Health Management

Laboratory data provides the foundation for predictive health management that identifies and addresses health issues before they become clinical problems. This proactive approach represents the future of personalized medicine and health optimization.

Early warning systems use lab trend analysis to identify emerging health issues before symptoms develop. Gradual changes in multiple related markers often predict health problems months or years before clinical diagnosis becomes possible.

Intervention timing optimization uses lab data to determine optimal timing for health interventions. Some interventions are most effective when implemented at specific stages of health decline or optimization, making timing crucial for success.

Prevention strategy personalization uses individual lab patterns and trends to customize prevention approaches. Generic prevention recommendations may be less effective than strategies tailored to individual risk patterns and metabolic characteristics.

Lifestyle-Laboratory Integration

Understanding relationships between lifestyle factors and laboratory results enables evidence-based lifestyle modifications that produce measurable health improvements. This integration transforms lifestyle choices from hopes into scientifically-guided interventions.

Exercise-lab correlations help optimize exercise prescriptions based on individual physiological responses. Different people respond differently to various exercise types and intensities, and lab markers can guide optimization of exercise programs.

Nutrition-lab relationships enable personalized nutrition strategies based on metabolic responses, nutrient status, and individual biochemistry. Generic nutrition recommendations may be less effective than approaches tailored to individual lab patterns.

Stress-lab connections reveal how stress management affects measurable health markers. Understanding individual stress responses helps optimize stress management strategies for maximum health benefit.

> *Lifestyle-Lab Integration Strategy Prompt: "Analyze how my lifestyle factors [describe diet, exercise, sleep, stress management] correlate with my lab value trends [provide relevant data]. What modifications might produce measurable improvements in my health markers?"*

Advanced Laboratory Interpretation Strategies

Functional Medicine Approach to Lab Analysis

Systems-Based Interpretation Framework

Functional medicine approaches laboratory interpretation from a systems perspective that examines root causes and interconnections rather than isolated abnormalities. This comprehensive approach often reveals optimization opportunities that conventional interpretation misses.

Root cause analysis uses lab patterns to identify underlying factors that affect multiple body systems simultaneously. For example, insulin resistance affects glucose metabolism, lipid patterns, inflammatory markers, and hormone production, creating recognizable patterns across seemingly unrelated tests.

Nutrient-function relationships examine how nutritional status affects cellular function and laboratory markers. Many lab abnormalities reflect nutritional insufficiencies rather than disease processes, making nutritional optimization a first-line intervention for many conditions.

Toxic burden assessment uses patterns of lab abnormalities to identify potential environmental exposures or toxic accumulations that affect health. Liver function tests, oxidative stress markers, and detoxification markers may reveal toxic burdens that conventional medicine overlooks.

Optimal Range Determination

Functional medicine typically uses tighter "optimal" ranges rather than broad "normal" ranges based on disease absence. These optimal ranges reflect values associated with excellent health and function rather than mere absence of pathology.

Age-specific optimization considers how optimal ranges change throughout life stages. Young adults may benefit from tighter optimal ranges that support peak performance, while older adults may have different optimization targets that balance function with realistic expectations.

Gender-specific considerations recognize that men and women have different optimal ranges for many markers due to hormonal, metabolic, and physiological differences. Using appropriate gender-specific targets improves the accuracy of optimization efforts.

Individual variation acknowledgment recognizes that some people naturally have optimal values outside population-based ranges. Establishing individual baselines and monitoring trends provides more meaningful information than comparing to population averages.

> *Functional Medicine Analysis Prompt: "Interpret my lab results [provide values] using functional medicine principles. What root cause*

factors might explain patterns in my results, and what optimal ranges should I target for my demographics and health goals?"

Specialty Laboratory Testing Considerations

Advanced Cardiovascular Assessment

Beyond basic lipid panels, advanced cardiovascular testing provides detailed information about heart disease risk that conventional testing cannot reveal. These specialized tests often identify high-risk individuals who appear normal on standard testing.

Advanced lipid analysis including LDL particle number, particle size, and apolipoprotein measurements provides more accurate cardiovascular risk assessment than basic cholesterol levels. Small, dense LDL particles are more dangerous than large, fluffy particles even at similar cholesterol concentrations.

Inflammatory marker assessment including high-sensitivity CRP, homocysteine, and other inflammatory markers reveals cardiovascular risk from inflammatory processes. Many heart attacks occur in people with normal cholesterol but elevated inflammatory markers.

Endothelial function testing measures the health of blood vessel walls, which affects cardiovascular risk independent of cholesterol levels. Tests like asymmetric dimethylarginine (ADMA) provide insights into vascular health that conventional testing misses.

Comprehensive Hormonal Assessment

Hormone testing requires understanding of timing, collection methods, and interpretation complexities that affect result accuracy and clinical utility. Many hormone tests are timing-dependent and require specific collection protocols.

Female hormone testing must account for menstrual cycle timing, contraceptive use, and life stage factors that dramatically affect hormone levels. Random hormone testing often provides misleading information about hormonal status and function.

Male hormone assessment includes not only total testosterone but also free testosterone, SHBG, estradiol, and other factors that affect hormonal function. Total testosterone alone provides incomplete information about male hormonal health.

Thyroid function assessment requires testing beyond basic TSH and T4 to include T3, reverse T3, and thyroid antibodies. Many people with thyroid symptoms have normal TSH but abnormal T3 conversion or autoimmune thyroid conditions.

> *Specialty Testing Research Prompt: "Research advanced testing options for [specific health concern] that might provide insights beyond standard laboratory panels. What specialized tests might be appropriate given my symptoms [describe] and risk factors [describe]?"*

Interpretation Challenges and Limitations

Understanding Test Limitations

Every laboratory test has limitations in sensitivity, specificity, and clinical utility that affect interpretation and decision-making. Understanding these limitations prevents over-reliance on individual test results and improves clinical decision-making.

False positive and false negative rates affect the reliability of test results, particularly for screening tests in low-prevalence conditions. Understanding predictive values helps interpret results appropriately based on individual risk factors.

Interference factors including medications, supplements, foods, and collection conditions can affect test results. Many people are unaware of factors that can cause misleading laboratory results, leading to inappropriate concern or missed opportunities for intervention.

Reference range limitations reflect the statistical and population-based nature of normal ranges rather than optimal health indicators. Understanding these limitations helps focus on trends and patterns rather than over-interpreting individual values.

Clinical Correlation Requirements

Laboratory results must always be interpreted in the context of clinical symptoms, physical examination findings, and individual health history. Lab values alone cannot diagnose conditions or guide treatment decisions without appropriate clinical correlation.

Symptom-lab disconnects occur when laboratory results don't correlate with clinical symptoms or expectations. These situations require careful evaluation of testing accuracy, timing, and alternative explanations rather than dismissing either symptoms or lab results.

Provider expertise requirements recognize that complex lab interpretation often requires specialized knowledge that may exceed primary care capabilities. Knowing when to seek subspecialty consultation improves diagnostic accuracy and treatment outcomes.

Transforming Laboratory Data into Health Optimization Intelligence

Understanding laboratory medicine beyond the simple "normal" versus "abnormal" classification transforms routine blood work from a passive medical procedure into an active tool for health optimization, disease prevention, and personalized wellness strategies. The comprehensive approach to lab interpretation outlined in this chapter provides you with the sophistication necessary to extract maximum value from your laboratory testing while working collaboratively with healthcare providers to achieve optimal health outcomes.

The knowledge you've gained about reference range limitations, demographic-specific optimal values, and systems-based interpretation enables you to identify optimization opportunities that conventional medical approaches routinely miss. When you understand that "normal" doesn't mean "optimal" and that trending patterns often provide more valuable information than individual results, you gain the ability to detect emerging health issues before they become clinical problems and implement interventions when they're most likely to be effective.

Your ability to interpret metabolic health markers with sophistication—understanding the progression from optimal glucose regulation through borderline prediabetes to insulin resistance—empowers you to implement preventive interventions at stages when they can still reverse metabolic dysfunction rather than merely managing established disease. This knowledge becomes particularly valuable given the epidemic of metabolic disorders that affects millions of people who remain unaware of their declining metabolic health until clinical diabetes or cardiovascular disease develops.

The AI-enhanced analysis frameworks and technology integration strategies provide you with tools to identify patterns and relationships in your laboratory data that even sophisticated healthcare providers might miss. When you can correlate lab trends with lifestyle factors, symptoms, and environmental influences, you gain insights into personalized optimization strategies that generic health recommendations cannot provide.

Your systematic approach to laboratory monitoring and provider communication transforms you from a passive recipient of medical opinions about your lab results into an informed participant in health optimization discussions. When you can present evidence-based requests for specific testing, discuss optimal ranges for your demographics, and communicate your health optimization goals clearly, you're more likely to receive collaborative care that supports your health objectives.

The comprehensive understanding of healthcare provider types and medical specialties from the previous chapter combines with your laboratory interpretation skills to ensure that you work with providers whose expertise matches your optimization needs. Some providers excel at pathology-focused medicine but may lack training in optimization approaches, while others specialize in functional medicine and optimization strategies. Matching your lab interpretation knowledge with appropriate provider expertise optimizes your healthcare outcomes. Remember that laboratory interpretation should always be done in collaboration with qualified healthcare providers who can integrate your test results with clinical examination findings, medical history, and individual risk factors. The goal is not to replace medical expertise but to become an informed partner who can contribute meaningfully to health optimization discussions and advocate effectively for comprehensive testing and interpretation that considers your complete health picture.

Your laboratory intelligence becomes the foundation for all other health optimization efforts outlined in this book. When you understand what your blood work actually reveals about your metabolic health, nutritional status, inflammatory burden, and organ function, you can implement targeted interventions with confidence and monitor their effectiveness objectively. This evidence-based approach to health optimization transforms hope-based wellness strategies into scientifically-guided interventions that produce measurable results.

The systematic approach to laboratory medicine outlined in this chapter represents a fundamental shift from reactive healthcare focused on treating disease after it develops to proactive health optimization that maintains excellent function and prevents disease development. This shift requires understanding laboratory medicine with the sophistication outlined in this chapter, but the investment in knowledge pays dividends in improved health outcomes, earlier problem detection, and more effective intervention strategies.

Your comprehensive laboratory intelligence now provides the foundation for the advanced health advocacy strategies outlined throughout this book, from combating healthcare bias to navigating medical specialties to building comprehensive health intelligence networks. When you understand what your laboratory results actually mean and can communicate that understanding effectively to healthcare providers, you possess a powerful tool for achieving optimal health outcomes that passive patients rarely experience.

The future of personalized medicine depends on individuals who understand their own health data with sufficient sophistication to participate meaningfully in optimization strategies. Your laboratory interpretation skills position you at the forefront of this healthcare evolution, where informed patients and collaborative providers work together to achieve health outcomes that conventional approaches cannot match.

Exercise 6.1 – Your Optimal Range Research

Pick one specific lab marker that's important for your health (vitamin D, ferritin, TSH, A1C, etc.). Research the functional medicine "optimal range" vs. the standard laboratory "normal range" for someone in your demographic.

Reflection: If your value is within "normal" range but outside "optimal" range, what would you want your provider to do about it?

Exercise 6.2 – Your Advanced Testing Wishlist

List the comprehensive lab tests you'd like to request but haven't. For each one, write WHY you want it and what decision the result would help you make.

Reflection: What stops you from asking for these tests? What would change if you asked anyway?

7

COMBAT HEALTHCARE GASLIGHTING AND DISMISSIVE CARE

When Healthcare Becomes Harmful

Medical gaslighting represents one of the most insidious forms of healthcare bias, where providers dismiss, minimize, or misattribute patient symptoms in ways that make patients question their own experiences and reality. Unlike simple medical errors or knowledge gaps, gaslighting involves a systematic undermining of patient credibility that can delay diagnosis, worsen health outcomes, and inflict lasting psychological harm.

The term "gaslighting" comes from the 1944 film "Gaslight," where a husband manipulates his wife into believing she's losing her sanity. In healthcare settings, gaslighting occurs when providers consistently dismiss patient concerns, attribute physical symptoms to psychological causes without investigation, or make patients feel foolish for seeking care. This behavior is particularly common when treating women, minorities, and patients with complex or poorly understood conditions.

Healthcare gaslighting isn't always intentional. Many providers operate under time pressure, algorithmic decision support, and training that may not adequately address healthcare disparities. However, the impact on patients is the same regardless of intent: delayed diagnoses, inadequate treatment, and erosion of trust in healthcare systems.

This chapter will teach you to recognize healthcare gaslighting patterns, document dismissive care systematically, build evidence-based responses to medical dismissal, and find healthcare providers who practice truly patient-centered care. You'll learn to protect your mental health while advocating for appropriate medical attention, and develop strategies for holding providers accountable when care falls below acceptable standards.

Recognizing Patterns of Medical Dismissal and Bias in Healthcare Interactions

Common Healthcare Gaslighting Phrases and Behaviors

Verbal Indicators of Medical Gaslighting

Healthcare gaslighting often follows predictable patterns. Learning to recognize these phrases helps you identify when dismissive care is occurring:

Direct Dismissal Phrases:

"It's All in Your Head." This dismissal reframes physical symptoms as psychological without proper evaluation.
"You're Too Young for That Condition." This response treats age as a diagnostic shortcut instead of investigating symptoms.
"Have You Considered Anxiety?" This question steers evaluation toward mental health without ruling out physical causes.

"Lose Weight and You'll Feel Better." This response uses weight to deflect from necessary diagnostic workup.
"Just Part of Being a Woman." This phrase normalizes severe symptoms instead of investigating them.
"Your Tests Are Normal." This response treats normal lab values as definitive when symptoms clearly indicate otherwise.
"You're Just Stressed." This attribution closes the door on investigation and places responsibility on the patient.

Subtle Gaslighting Techniques:

Interrupting Symptom Descriptions. Interrupting or cutting off symptom descriptions prevents full clinical picture from emerging.
Mental Health Focus Without Physical Workup. Focusing on mental health without investigating physical causes is a common form of dismissal.
Condescending Language. Using condescending language or tone signals that the provider does not view you as a partner.
Dismissing Research or Questions. Dismissing patient research or questions discourages informed participation in care.
Oversimplified Attribution. Attributing complex symptoms to simple explanations without investigation often misses real conditions.
Shaming for Seeking Care. Making patients feel foolish for seeking care discourages future advocacy.

Behavioral Patterns of Dismissive Care

Time Minimization: Providers who consistently rush through appointments without adequate symptom exploration **Question Avoidance:** Providers who deflect or ignore direct questions about diagnosis and treatment **Defensive Responses:** Providers who become defensive when patients advocate for themselves or ask for second opinions **Paternalistic Decision-Making:** Providers who make treatment decisions without meaningful patient input or explanation

Gaslighting Recognition Prompt: "Help me analyze this healthcare interaction for potential gaslighting or dismissive behavior: [describe interaction]. What patterns suggest inappropriate dismissal of my concerns, and how should I respond?"

Demographic-Specific Gaslighting Patterns

Gender-Based Medical Gaslighting

Women face unique patterns of medical dismissal that reflect broader societal biases:

Pain Minimization: Women's pain reports are more likely to be attributed to emotional causes or considered exaggerated **Hormonal Attribution**: Complex symptoms dismissed as hormonal issues without investigation **Appearance-Based Assumptions**: Weight, age, or appearance used to dismiss legitimate health concerns **Reproductive Health Reductionism**: All health issues attributed to reproductive system without comprehensive evaluation

Racial and Ethnic Healthcare Gaslighting

Patients of color face systematic dismissal patterns rooted in historical medical racism:

Pain Underestimation: Persistent myths about pain tolerance leading to inadequate pain management **Stereotype-Based Assumptions**: Health behaviors assumed based on racial stereotypes rather than individual assessment **Language Barriers Exploitation**: Communication difficulties used to avoid thorough evaluation **Socioeconomic Dismissal**: Health concerns attributed to socioeconomic factors without medical investigation

Age-Based Healthcare Dismissal

Young Adult Dismissal: Serious conditions dismissed because "you're too young" **Older Adult Ageism**: Symptoms attributed to normal aging without investigation **Middle-Age Minimization**: Women's symptoms during perimenopause attributed solely to hormonal changes

Identifying Systemic vs. Individual Gaslighting

Provider-Level Gaslighting

Individual providers who consistently engage in dismissive behavior patterns:

Repeated Dismissal. Repeated dismissal across multiple appointments indicates a pattern, not an isolated interaction.
Defensive Responses. Defensive responses to patient advocacy signal unwillingness to engage collaboratively.
Closed to Alternatives. Unwillingness to consider alternative diagnoses locks care into a single assumption.
Inadequate Care Patterns. Documented patterns of inadequate care warrant formal review and a change of provider.

System-Level Gaslighting

Institutional practices that systematically dismiss patient concerns:

Efficiency-First Protocols. Protocols that prioritize efficiency over thorough evaluation embed dismissal into the system.
Bias-Reinforcing Algorithms. Algorithmic decision support that reinforces bias shapes care in ways providers may not notice.
Inadequate Bias Training. Training programs that inadequately address healthcare disparities leave providers unprepared to recognize bias.
Misaligned Financial Incentives. Financial incentives that discourage comprehensive evaluation work against patient interests.

System Analysis Prompt: "Help me determine whether the dismissive care I'm experiencing is primarily from individual providers or systemic healthcare issues. Based on my experiences [provide details], what patterns suggest institutional versus individual problems?"

Using AI to Validate Your Health Concerns and Research Supporting Evidence

Evidence-Based Validation Strategies

Symptom Validation Research

When providers dismiss your concerns, use AI to research evidence that validates your experiences:

Symptom Validation Prompt: "Research medical literature that validates these symptoms [describe symptoms] as legitimate medical concerns. Find studies that show these symptoms warrant investigation, particularly in [your demographic], and identify conditions that commonly present with this symptom pattern."

Demographic-Specific Research

Research how your symptoms present in your specific demographic to counter dismissive assumptions:

Demographic Research Prompt: "Find research on how [specific condition or symptoms] present in [your demographic characteristics]. What studies show that these symptoms are often dismissed or misdiagnosed in people like me, and what evidence supports the need for comprehensive evaluation?"

Building Evidence-Based Responses to Dismissal

Constructing Professional Responses to Gaslighting

When facing medical dismissal, prepare evidence-based responses that redirect conversation toward appropriate care:

Response to "It's all in your head": "Recent research shows that [cite specific studies] patients with my symptom pattern often have underlying medical conditions that require investigation. I'd like to discuss ruling out these medical causes before considering psychological factors."

Response to "You're too young for that condition": "While this condition is more common in older patients, studies show it does occur in younger people, particularly those with [your risk factors]. Could we discuss age-appropriate screening approaches?"

Response to "Your tests are normal": "I understand these initial tests are normal, but research indicates that [cite relevant studies] additional testing may be needed for patients with persistent symptoms like mine. What would be the next appropriate step in evaluation?"

> *Response Development Prompt: "Help me develop professional, evidence-based responses to these dismissive statements from my healthcare provider: [list specific dismissive comments]. Include relevant research citations and redirect toward appropriate medical investigation."*

Research Documentation for Medical Advocacy

Creating Evidence Portfolios

Compile research evidence that supports your need for appropriate medical care:

Symptom Validation Research: Studies showing your symptoms warrant medical investigation **Diagnostic Approach Research:** Evidence for comprehensive evaluation approaches **Condition-Specific Research:** Information about conditions that might explain your symptoms **Healthcare Disparity Research:** Studies documenting bias in your demographic

Medical Literature Integration

Learn to effectively integrate medical research into healthcare conversations:

Cite Specific Studies. Cite specific studies rather than general information to ground your advocacy in evidence.
Peer-Reviewed Focus. Focus on peer-reviewed research from reputable medical journals rather than popular articles.
Demographic Relevance. Emphasize research relevant to your specific demographic to show why standard criteria may not apply.
Collaborative Framing. Present research as collaborative information sharing rather than confrontational challenge.

Building Credible Medical Arguments to Counter Dismissive Healthcare Providers

Strategic Medical Argumentation

Evidence-Based Advocacy Framework

Clinical Justification: Using medical standards to support your requests

Reference Clinical Guidelines. Reference clinical guidelines that support comprehensive evaluation for your presentation.
Cite Thorough Diagnostic Evidence. Cite medical literature showing benefits of thorough diagnostic approaches.

Document Criteria Fulfillment. Document how current symptoms meet criteria for further investigation.
Present Risk Factors. Present family history and risk factors that justify additional testing.

Professional Communication Strategy

Frame your advocacy in professional medical language:

Guideline-Based Framing. "Based on clinical guidelines for [condition], what evaluation approach would you recommend?"
Differential Framing. "Given my symptom pattern and family history, what differential diagnoses should we consider?"
Research-Based Framing. "Research suggests that patients with my presentation benefit from [specific evaluation]. How can we implement this approach?"

> *Medical Argument Development Prompt: "Help me build a professional medical argument for why my symptoms [describe symptoms] warrant comprehensive evaluation. Include relevant clinical guidelines, research evidence, and professional language that encourages collaborative problem-solving."*

Overcoming Common Dismissal Tactics

Systematic Responses to Dismissive Statements

When told "Let's wait and see": Research-based response: "Studies show that early intervention for [relevant conditions] leads to better outcomes. Given my symptom progression and family history, what specific timeline and monitoring criteria would you recommend? What symptoms would prompt immediate evaluation?"

When symptoms are attributed to stress: Evidence-based response: "I understand stress can affect health, but research indicates we should rule out medical causes before attributing symptoms to psychological factors. What tests would help us distinguish between medical and stress-related causes?"

When told tests are "unnecessary": Guidelines-based response: "According to [specific medical guidelines], patients with my presentation typically receive [specific evaluation]. Could you help me understand why this approach might not be appropriate in my case?"

Documentation and Accountability Strategies

Creating Records of Dismissive Care

Interaction Documentation:

Time and Provider Details. Record date, time, and provider information for all dismissive interactions.
Exact Quotes. Capture exact quotes of dismissive statements or behaviors.
Witness Information. Note any witnesses present during interactions who can corroborate.
Tests and Treatments Denied. Document specific tests or treatments requested and denied.
Provider Reasoning. Record the provider's stated reasoning for denial or dismissal as given.

Medical Record Documentation:

Request Provider Notes. Request copies of all provider notes from appointments for your records.
Review for Accuracy. Review notes for accuracy and appropriate documentation of your concerns.

Identify Discrepancies. Identify discrepancies between your experience and provider documentation.
Document Omissions. Document when important symptoms or concerns are omitted from medical records.

> *Documentation Strategy Prompt: "Help me create a systematic approach to documenting dismissive healthcare interactions. What information should I record, and how can I organize this documentation to support advocacy efforts or potential complaints?"*

Finding Healthcare Providers Who Practice Patient-Centered Care

Provider Research and Evaluation

Identifying Patient-Centered Providers

Research Strategies for Provider Selection:

Equity-Trained Providers. Look for professional training that includes healthcare equity and bias awareness.
Continuing Disparity Education. Look for participation in continuing education about healthcare disparities.
Published Patient-Centered Work. Look for published work or presentations on patient-centered care.
Advocacy-Focused Affiliations. Look for hospital or clinic affiliations with patient advocacy focus.
Respectful Communication Reviews. Look for patient reviews that specifically mention respectful communication and thorough evaluation.

Interview Questions for Potential Providers

Use specific questions to evaluate whether providers practice truly patient-centered care:

Patient Research Approach. "How do you approach patients who have done research about their symptoms?"
Experience with Your Condition. "What's your experience treating [your condition/demographics]?"
Unresolved Symptoms Approach. "How do you handle situations where initial tests don't explain persistent symptoms?"
Shared Decision-Making Approach. "What's your approach to shared decision-making with patients?"
Disparity Research Currency. "How do you stay current with research on healthcare disparities?"

> *Provider Evaluation Prompt: "Help me develop interview questions and evaluation criteria for finding healthcare providers who practice patient-centered care. Focus on identifying providers who would be appropriate for someone with my health profile [describe relevant factors]."*

Building Relationships with Quality Providers

Establishing Collaborative Provider Relationships

Initial Appointment Strategy:

Prepare Health History. Prepare comprehensive health history and current concerns before the first visit.
Bring Research and Questions. Bring research and questions that demonstrate informed participation.
Communicate Collaboration Preferences. Clearly communicate your preferences for collaborative care early in the relationship.

Assess Provider Response. Assess provider response to your preparation and advocacy to evaluate fit.

Long-Term Relationship Development:

Regular Goal Communication. Maintain regular communication about health goals and concerns.
Shared Decision-Making. Practice shared decision-making about treatment approaches over time.
Ongoing Condition Education. Continue ongoing education about your conditions and preferences together.
Care Quality Feedback. Provide feedback about care quality and communication effectiveness.

Alternative and Integrative Care Options

Exploring Comprehensive Care Approaches

Functional Medicine Providers: Practitioners who focus on root cause analysis and comprehensive evaluation **Integrative Medicine:** Providers who combine conventional and evidence-based complementary approaches **Naturopathic Medicine:** Licensed practitioners with training in natural treatment approaches **Direct Primary Care:** Subscription-based primary care that allows longer appointment times

Evaluating Alternative Providers

Research credentials and approaches of alternative providers:

Licensing and Certifications. Verify professional licensing and board certifications before engaging alternative providers.
Accredited Training. Confirm training from accredited institutions.
Evidence-Based Practices. Evaluate evidence-based practice approaches in their work.

Integration with Conventional Care. Look for integration with conventional medical care when appropriate.
Patient Safety Protocols. Review patient safety protocols and referral practices.

> *Alternative Care Research Prompt: "Research [specific type of alternative provider] options in my area. What credentials should I look for, and how can I evaluate whether these providers practice evidence-based medicine and maintain appropriate safety standards?"*

Legal and Advocacy Resources for Medical Malpractice and Bias Cases

Understanding Legal Protections and Options

Patient Rights and Legal Standards

Standard of Care Violations: When provider behavior falls below accepted medical standards **Informed Consent Violations:** When providers fail to provide adequate information for decision-making **Discrimination and Bias:** When care differs based on protected characteristics rather than medical factors **Emergency Care Violations:** When emergency departments fail to provide appropriate screening and stabilization

Documentation for Legal Protection

Legal-Standard Documentation:

Chronological Interaction Records. Maintain detailed chronological records of all medical interactions.
Complete Records Copies. Keep copies of all medical records and test results.

Harm Documentation. Document specific harm resulting from inadequate care.
Witness Statements. Collect witness statements when available to corroborate your account.
Bias or Discrimination Evidence. Preserve evidence of provider bias or discrimination for potential action.

> *Legal Documentation Prompt: "Help me understand what documentation would be necessary to support a legal complaint about inadequate healthcare. What specific information should I maintain, and how should I organize it for potential legal review?"*

Professional Accountability Resources

Medical Board Complaints

When provider behavior violates professional standards:

State Licensing Board Process. Research state medical licensing board complaint processes in your jurisdiction.
Documentation Requirements. Understand documentation requirements for professional misconduct complaints.
Filing Timeline. Know the timeline requirements for filing complaints so you don't miss deadlines.
Outcomes and Limitations. Understand potential outcomes and limitations of medical board actions before filing.

Healthcare System Accountability

Internal Complaint Processes:

Patient Relations Departments. File through hospital patient relations departments for communication issues.

Quality Committees. Escalate to medical staff quality committees for clinical concerns.
Risk Management. Contact risk management departments for incidents with potential liability.
Internal Patient Advocacy. Use patient advocacy services within healthcare systems where available.

External Oversight:

State Health Department. File with state health department oversight for serious care issues.
Joint Commission. File Joint Commission complaints for accredited hospitals.
Insurer Quality Programs. Report to insurance company provider quality programs when warranted.
Professional Ethics Committees. File with professional organization ethics committees for ethical violations.

Patient Advocacy and Support Resources

Professional Patient Advocacy Services

Independent Patient Advocates: Professional advocates who can attend appointments and support healthcare navigation **Legal Patient Advocates:** Attorneys specializing in healthcare rights and medical malpractice **Medical Advocates:** Healthcare professionals who provide independent consultation and advocacy **Specialized Advocates:** Advocates with expertise in specific conditions or demographics

Community and Organizational Support

Disease-Specific Organizations: Patient advocacy groups focused on specific conditions **Healthcare Equity Organizations:** Groups working to address healthcare disparities **Legal Aid Organizations**: Non-profit legal services for healthcare access issues **Community Health Centers:** Healthcare providers with explicit health equity focus

> *Advocacy Resource Research Prompt: "Research patient advocacy resources available for [specific situation/condition/demographic]. What organizations or services could provide support for healthcare quality issues, and how can I access these resources?"*

Protecting Your Mental Health While Advocating for Medical Care

Psychological Impact of Medical Gaslighting

Understanding Gaslighting Trauma

Medical gaslighting can cause significant psychological harm:

Self-Doubt. Self-doubt about symptom validity and severity is a common psychological effect of gaslighting.
Medical Care Anxiety. Anxiety about seeking medical care can develop after repeated dismissive encounters.
Depression from Dismissal. Depression can develop from repeatedly feeling unheard or dismissed.
Medical PTSD. Post-traumatic stress from medical encounters is a documented consequence of serious gaslighting.
Erosion of Trust. Erosion of trust in healthcare systems can persist long after the original incident.

Validation and Recovery Strategies

Self-Validation Techniques:

Symptom Journals. Keep detailed symptom journals to validate your experiences against dismissal.
Connecting with Others. Connect with others who have similar experiences to normalize your reality.
Patient-Centered Validation. Seek validation from healthcare providers who practice patient-centered care.
Research-Based Validation. Use research to confirm that your symptoms warrant investigation.

Mental Health Support Integration

Therapeutic Support: Working with mental health professionals who understand medical trauma **Support Groups**: Connecting with others who have experienced healthcare dismissal **Advocacy Communities**: Participating in patient advocacy organizations **Professional Consultation**: Seeking independent medical opinions to validate concerns

> *Mental Health Support Planning Prompt: "Help me develop strategies to protect my mental health while advocating for appropriate medical care. What approaches can help me maintain confidence in my symptoms and experiences while dealing with dismissive healthcare providers?"*

Building Resilience for Healthcare Advocacy

Emotional Preparation Strategies

Pre-Appointment Preparation:

Review Research for Confidence. Review research and documentation to build confidence before the appointment.

Prepare Responses. Prepare responses to potential dismissive statements in advance.

Bring Support People. Bring support people when appropriate to witness and back you up.

Post-Appointment Self-Care. Plan self-care activities after potentially difficult appointments.

During-Appointment Strategies:

Stay Fact-Focused. Stay focused on facts and documentation rather than emotional responses in the moment.

Request Written Documentation. Request written documentation of provider recommendations or dismissals.

Take Notes or Bring Help. Take notes or bring someone to help remember important information.

Leave if Necessary. Leave appointments early if provider behavior becomes inappropriate.

Post-Appointment Recovery:

Debrief with Support. Debrief with supportive friends or family members after difficult appointments.

Review and Reflect. Review what went well and what could be improved for next time.

Plan Next Steps. Plan next steps for continued advocacy based on what happened.

Restorative Self-Care. Engage in self-care activities that restore emotional balance.

Advanced Strategies for Overcoming Systematic Dismissal

Systemic Advocacy Approaches

Pattern Documentation for Systemic Change

Individual Case Building: Documenting patterns of dismissive care for potential legal or regulatory action **Community Advocacy**: Working with other patients to document systematic problems **Research Participation**: Contributing to studies documenting healthcare disparities **Policy Advocacy**: Supporting legislative or regulatory changes that address healthcare bias

Creating Accountability Networks

Professional Network Development

Provider Accountability: Building relationships with healthcare providers who hold colleagues accountable **Administrative Advocacy**: Working with healthcare administrators to address systematic bias **Educational Advocacy**: Contributing to healthcare professional education about bias and patient advocacy **Community Leadership**: Leading community efforts to improve healthcare quality and equity

Reclaiming Your Voice in Healthcare

Combat healthcare gaslighting requires both individual resilience and systematic advocacy strategies. By learning to recognize dismissive care patterns, building evidence-based responses, and finding truly patient-centered providers, you protect yourself from harmful medical encounters while advocating for appropriate care.

The strategies outlined in this chapter provide both defensive and offensive approaches to medical gaslighting. Defensive strategies protect your mental health and maintain confidence in your experiences, while offensive strategies actively challenge dismissive care and hold providers accountable for appropriate professional behavior.

Remember that healthcare gaslighting reflects systemic problems within healthcare rather than personal failings on your part. Your symptoms are real, your concerns are valid, and you deserve respectful, comprehensive medical care. The advocacy skills you develop in response to dismissive care become powerful tools for achieving better health outcomes and contributing to healthcare system improvements.

Your ability to recognize and respond to healthcare gaslighting protects not only your own health but also contributes to broader efforts to improve healthcare quality and equity. Every time you successfully advocate for appropriate care, you create precedents and relationships that can benefit other patients facing similar challenges.

The comprehensive approach to combating healthcare gaslighting outlined in this chapter transforms you from a vulnerable patient into a resilient advocate who cannot be easily dismissed or marginalized within healthcare systems. This resilience becomes the foundation for all other healthcare advocacy efforts and ensures that your voice remains strong and credible in all medical interactions.

Exercise 7.1 – Your Gaslighting Inventory

Write down every dismissive phrase a healthcare provider has ever said to you. Don't sanitize or excuse them. Then next to each one, write how you wish you'd responded in the moment.

Reflection: *Which of these phrases still echoes in your head and affects how you approach healthcare today?*

Exercise 7.2 – Your Response Playbook

Using the response strategies from this chapter, write out exactly what you'll say the next time a provider dismisses you. Practice it out loud. Bring this page to your next appointment.

Reflection: *What outcome are you afraid of if you push back? What outcome are you afraid of if you don't?*

8

NAVIGATING MISDIAGNOSIS - WHEN HEALTHCARE GETS IT WRONG

The Hidden Epidemic of Medical Errors

Twelve million Americans are misdiagnosed every year—a staggering statistic that represents one in twenty patients receiving incorrect, delayed, or missed diagnoses that can fundamentally alter their health outcomes. For women, minorities, and patients with complex symptoms, these numbers climb even higher, reflecting systematic biases in diagnostic processes that can mean the difference between early intervention and years of unnecessary suffering.

Misdiagnosis isn't simply a matter of medical complexity or rare conditions confounding well-meaning providers. It represents a failure of healthcare systems that rely on pattern recognition trained on biased data, algorithmic decision support that perpetuates historical disparities, and diagnostic protocols that assume male, white, middle-aged presentations as the standard. When your symptoms don't fit these narrow parameters, misdiagnosis becomes not just possible but probable.

The three types of diagnostic errors—missed diagnosis (failure to identify a condition), delayed diagnosis (correct diagnosis made too late), and incorrect diagnosis (wrong condition identified)—each carry distinct challenges for patient advocacy. A missed diagnosis means your real condition remains untreated while you suffer in medical limbo. A delayed diagnosis allows treatable conditions to progress unnecessarily, sometimes beyond the point of optimal intervention. An incorrect diagnosis subjects you to inappropriate treatments while your actual condition worsens.

Understanding misdiagnosis patterns empowers you to recognize when diagnostic errors might be occurring, research alternative explanations for persistent symptoms, and advocate strategically for reconsideration of diagnostic conclusions. This chapter will teach you to identify red flags suggesting misdiagnosis, use AI tools to research alternative diagnoses, challenge diagnostic conclusions professionally, and navigate the complex process of seeking accurate medical evaluation when initial diagnoses prove inadequate.

Recognizing the Red Flags of Potential Misdiagnosis

Understanding Diagnostic Error Patterns

Common Misdiagnosis Scenarios

Diagnostic errors follow predictable patterns that you can learn to recognize:

Anchoring Bias in Diagnosis: Providers focus on initial impressions and fail to consider alternatives when new information emerges. Your chest pain gets labeled as anxiety because you're a young woman, even when cardiac testing hasn't been completed.

Pattern Recognition Failures: Conditions that present atypically in your demographic get misdiagnosed as more "common" conditions. Your autoimmune disease gets diagnosed as depression because fatigue and joint pain in young women are often attributed to psychological causes.

Diagnostic Momentum: Once a diagnosis enters your medical record, subsequent providers accept it without independent evaluation. Your irritable bowel syndrome diagnosis from five years ago prevents adequate evaluation of new abdominal symptoms that might indicate inflammatory bowel disease.

Premature Closure: Providers reach diagnostic conclusions without adequate investigation. Your heavy menstrual bleeding gets attributed to stress without evaluation for fibroids, endometriosis, or bleeding disorders.

> *Misdiagnosis Pattern Recognition Prompt: "Based on my diagnostic history [provide timeline of diagnoses and treatments], what patterns might suggest misdiagnosis? What red flags indicate that my symptoms weren't adequately investigated?"*

Symptom-Treatment Mismatch Recognition

When Treatment Doesn't Work as Expected

One of the clearest indicators of potential misdiagnosis is persistent symptoms despite appropriate treatment:

Treatment Resistance Patterns: You've followed treatment recommendations faithfully, but symptoms persist or worsen. Your "acid reflux" doesn't respond to proton pump inhibitors because you actually have gastroparesis.

Symptom Expansion Despite Treatment: New symptoms develop while you're being treated for your diagnosed condition. Your "fibromyalgia" treatment doesn't prevent new neurological symptoms that might indicate multiple sclerosis.

Side Effects That Seem Disproportionate: Treatment side effects seem unusually severe or don't match expected responses. Your antidepressant causes cardiac symptoms because your "depression" is actually a thyroid condition.

Cyclical Treatment Failures: You experience temporary improvement followed by symptom return, suggesting the underlying cause wasn't addressed. Your "sinus infections" keep recurring because you actually have allergic rhinitis or structural abnormalities.

Timeline Analysis for Diagnostic Accuracy

Reviewing Your Diagnostic Journey

Systematic analysis of your diagnostic timeline can reveal patterns suggesting misdiagnosis:

Rapid Diagnosis Red Flags: Diagnoses reached very quickly without comprehensive evaluation often reflect bias rather than thorough investigation. Complex symptom clusters attributed to single explanations without ruling out alternatives.

Diagnostic Inconsistencies: Different providers reaching different conclusions about the same symptoms. Your fatigue gets diagnosed as chronic fatigue syndrome by one provider and depression by another, suggesting neither conducted adequate evaluation.

Symptom Timeline Mismatches: Your diagnosed condition doesn't explain the timeline or progression of your symptoms. Your "osteoarthritis" pain began suddenly rather than gradually, suggesting alternative explanations.

Timeline Analysis Prompt: "Analyze my diagnostic timeline: [provide chronological list of symptoms, diagnoses, and treatments]. What inconsistencies suggest misdiagnosis, and what alternative diagnostic approaches should I consider?"

Using AI to Research Alternative Diagnoses and Validate Symptoms

Comprehensive Symptom Research Strategies

Multi-Source Diagnostic Research

When you suspect misdiagnosis, systematic research becomes critical for identifying alternative explanations:

Symptom Cluster Analysis: Use AI to research conditions that explain your complete symptom pattern rather than isolated symptoms:

Alternative Diagnosis Research Prompt: "I was diagnosed with [current diagnosis] but have these persisting symptoms: [comprehensive symptom list with timeline]. What conditions better explain this complete symptom pattern, particularly in someone with my demographics [age, gender, ethnicity]?"

Demographic-Specific Presentation Research: Many conditions present differently across demographics, leading to misdiagnosis when providers expect textbook presentations:

Demographic Presentation Prompt: "Research how [suspected condition] presents in [your demographic characteristics]. What symptoms are commonly missed when providers expect typical presentations, and what diagnostic criteria are most appropriate for people like me?"

Comorbidity Pattern Analysis: Some conditions commonly occur together, and missing one can lead to inadequate treatment of both:

Comorbidity Research Prompt: "Given my diagnosed condition [current diagnosis] and persistent symptoms [list symptoms], what conditions commonly co-occur with my diagnosis that might explain my ongoing health issues?"

Evidence-Based Diagnostic Validation

Research-Supported Symptom Validation

When providers dismiss symptoms as psychological or normal, use research to validate their medical significance:

Symptom Legitimacy Research: Find studies documenting that your symptoms represent legitimate medical concerns requiring investigation:

Symptom Validation Prompt: "Find peer-reviewed research showing that these symptoms [list specific symptoms] warrant medical investigation and are not 'normal' or purely psychological, particularly in [your demographic]."

Biomarker and Diagnostic Criteria Research: Research objective measures that support alternative diagnoses:

Diagnostic Criteria Prompt: "Research diagnostic criteria for [suspected condition] and identify objective tests, biomarkers, or assessments that could confirm or rule out this diagnosis in someone with my symptom pattern."

Treatment Response Research: Use treatment response patterns to support diagnostic reconsideration:

> *Treatment Response Analysis Prompt: "Research why someone with [current diagnosis] might not respond to standard treatments [list tried treatments] and what alternative diagnoses might explain this treatment resistance."*

International and Alternative Diagnostic Approaches

Expanding Diagnostic Perspectives

Different healthcare systems and medical traditions may offer alternative diagnostic frameworks:

International Diagnostic Standards: Research how other countries approach your symptoms or condition:

> *International Standards Research Prompt: "Compare diagnostic approaches for [symptoms/condition] between US medical practice and other healthcare systems. What alternative diagnostic criteria or treatment approaches might be more appropriate for my presentation?"*

Integrative Medicine Perspectives: Functional and integrative medicine often identify root causes that conventional medicine misses:

> *Integrative Approach Research Prompt: "Research how functional medicine or integrative medicine approaches [my symptoms/condition]. What root cause analyses or diagnostic approaches might explain my symptoms better than my current diagnosis?"*

Building Evidence-Based Cases for Diagnostic Reconsideration

Strategic Diagnostic Challenge Framework

Professional Diagnostic Questioning

Challenging a diagnosis requires strategic communication that encourages provider reconsideration without creating defensive responses:

Evidence-Based Diagnostic Discussion: Present research and symptom analysis systematically:

"I've been researching my symptoms and found studies showing that [specific symptoms] can indicate [alternative condition], particularly in [my demographic]. Given that my current treatment isn't providing expected results, could we discuss whether additional diagnostic evaluation might be appropriate?"

Timeline Presentation Strategy: Organize your diagnostic journey to highlight inconsistencies:

"Looking at my symptom timeline, I notice that [specific observation about timing/progression] doesn't align with typical patterns for [current diagnosis]. Research suggests this pattern might be more consistent with [alternative condition]. What additional evaluation would help clarify this?"

Treatment Response Documentation: Use treatment failures as diagnostic evidence:

"After [time period] of treatment for [current diagnosis] with [list treatments], my symptoms haven't improved as expected. Studies show that treatment resistance in [current diagnosis] might suggest [alternative conditions]. What diagnostic approaches could help distinguish between these possibilities?"

Diagnostic Challenge Prompt: "Help me prepare a professional, evidence-based presentation challenging my diagnosis of [current diagnosis]. Include research supporting alternative diagnoses and specific requests for additional evaluation that demonstrate collaborative problem-solving."

Second Opinion Strategy Development

Strategic Provider Selection for Alternative Evaluation

Different Healthcare System Selection: Choose providers from different healthcare systems to avoid confirmation bias and shared protocols:

"I'm seeking evaluation at [different healthcare system] because I want an independent assessment of my symptoms without influence from my current medical records or previous diagnostic assumptions."

Specialist Expertise Matching: Research specialists who have specific expertise in alternative diagnoses you're considering:

Specialist Selection Prompt: "Research specialists in [geographic area] who have expertise in [alternative conditions I'm considering]. What credentials, research experience, or patient populations suggest these providers would be appropriate for independent diagnostic evaluation?"

Academic Medical Center Consultation: Teaching hospitals often provide more comprehensive evaluation:

"Academic medical centers typically have access to the latest diagnostic approaches and may be more willing to consider complex or unusual presentations that community providers might miss."

Diagnostic Documentation and Evidence Building

Comprehensive Diagnostic Portfolio Development

Systematic Documentation Strategy: Create comprehensive documentation that supports diagnostic reconsideration:

Complete Symptom Timeline: Detailed chronological documentation of symptom development, changes, and responses to treatment **Treatment Response Records:** Documentation of all attempted treatments, adherence, and outcomes **Research Summary:** Professional summary of research supporting alternative diagnostic considerations **Family History Relevance:** Analysis of family health patterns that support alternative diagnoses **Functional Impact Assessment:** Documentation of how symptoms affect daily life in ways not explained by current diagnosis

> *Diagnostic Portfolio Prompt: "Help me organize my medical information into a comprehensive diagnostic portfolio that supports reconsideration of my diagnosis. What documentation most effectively demonstrates the need for additional evaluation?"*

Navigating Multiple Provider Opinions and Conflicting Diagnoses

Managing Diagnostic Disagreement

Systematic Approach to Conflicting Medical Opinions

When different providers reach different diagnostic conclusions, strategic analysis becomes essential:

Opinion Evaluation Framework: Analyze conflicting diagnoses systematically:

Conflicting Opinion Analysis Prompt: "I've received different diagnoses from different providers: Provider A diagnosed [diagnosis 1], Provider B diagnosed [diagnosis 2], and Provider C diagnosed [diagnosis 3]. Help me evaluate the evidence base for each diagnosis and develop questions that might help clarify which is most accurate."

Expertise Assessment: Evaluate whether provider expertise matches your condition complexity:

"My primary care physician diagnosed [condition], but my specialist suggests [different condition]. Given my symptom pattern [describe], which provider's expertise is most relevant to making an accurate diagnosis?"

Testing and Evidence Integration: Use diagnostic testing to resolve conflicting opinions:

"Different providers have reached different conclusions about my symptoms. What diagnostic tests would provide objective evidence to distinguish between [list competing diagnoses]?"

Third Opinion Strategy

When Two Opinions Aren't Enough

Sometimes additional perspectives provide diagnostic clarity:

Academic Specialist Consultation: Seek evaluation from providers who specialize in complex diagnostic cases:

Third Opinion Strategy Prompt: "I've received conflicting diagnoses of [list diagnoses] from different providers. What type of specialist or medical center would be most appropriate for a definitive diagnostic evaluation of my symptom pattern?"

Multidisciplinary Evaluation: Some medical centers offer team-based diagnostic approaches:

"Multidisciplinary clinics that include several specialists evaluating patients together can provide more comprehensive diagnostic assessment than individual provider consultations."

Collaborative Diagnostic Resolution

Working with Providers to Reach Accurate Diagnosis

Shared Decision-Making in Diagnostic Uncertainty: When diagnosis remains uncertain, work with providers to develop systematic approaches:

"Given that my diagnosis remains uncertain, could we develop a systematic plan for ruling out the most concerning possibilities and monitoring for diagnostic clarification over time?"

Treatment Trial as Diagnostic Tool: Sometimes treatment responses help clarify diagnoses:

"Since we're considering both [condition A] and [condition B], would a trial of [specific treatment] help distinguish between these possibilities based on treatment response?"

Timeline-Based Diagnostic Approach: Establish clear criteria for diagnostic reconsideration:

"If my symptoms don't improve with treatment for [current diagnosis] within [specific timeframe], what alternative diagnoses should we consider, and what additional evaluation would be appropriate?"

Advocating for Comprehensive Re-evaluation

Systematic Re-evaluation Request Strategy

Medical Justification for Diagnostic Reconsideration

Clinical Guidelines Supporting Re-evaluation: Research medical guidelines that support comprehensive diagnostic reconsideration:

> *Re-evaluation Research Prompt: "Research clinical guidelines that support diagnostic reconsideration when patients have [my specific situation - treatment resistance, symptom progression, etc.]. What evidence-based criteria justify comprehensive re-evaluation?"*

Quality Assurance Standards: Frame diagnostic reconsideration as quality assurance:

"Medical quality standards recommend diagnostic reconsideration when treatment outcomes don't meet expectations. Given my ongoing symptoms despite treatment, comprehensive re-evaluation aligns with quality care principles."

Patient Safety Considerations: Position diagnostic accuracy as patient safety issue:

"Accurate diagnosis is fundamental to patient safety. My persistent symptoms despite treatment suggest the need for diagnostic reconsideration to ensure I receive appropriate care."

Advanced Diagnostic Testing Advocacy

Comprehensive Testing Request Strategy

Evidence-Based Testing Requests: Use research to support requests for comprehensive diagnostic workup:

> *Testing Advocacy Prompt: "Based on my symptoms [list] and treatment resistance [describe], what diagnostic tests would comprehensive medical guidelines recommend to rule out alternative diagnoses? What evidence supports the medical necessity of these tests?"*

Specialist Referral Justification: Build cases for specialist evaluation:

"Given the complexity of my symptom pattern and diagnostic uncertainty, specialist evaluation would provide expertise in differential diagnosis that's beyond the scope of primary care."

Timeline Urgency Communication: When appropriate, communicate urgency for diagnostic resolution:

"My symptoms are progressively affecting my function and quality of life. Timely diagnostic resolution is important for preventing further deterioration and optimizing treatment outcomes."

Documentation Strategies for Misdiagnosis Cases

Legal and Medical Record Management

Systematic Documentation for Accountability

Comprehensive Interaction Documentation: Maintain detailed records of all diagnostic interactions:

Provider Statement Documentation: Record exact quotes about diagnostic reasoning and decision-making **Test Request and Denial Documentation:** Document what testing was requested, approved, denied, and provider reasoning **Treatment Response Documentation:** Systematic tracking of treatment attempts, adherence, and outcomes **Symptom Progression Documentation:** Detailed tracking of symptom changes over time despite treatment

> *Documentation Strategy Prompt: "Create a systematic documentation framework for tracking my diagnostic journey that could support requests for re-evaluation or potential accountability issues. What information is most important to document consistently?"*

Evidence Portfolio for Provider Communication

Professional Medical Communication Documentation

Research Integration Documentation: Maintain professional summaries of research supporting diagnostic reconsideration:

Peer-Reviewed Literature Summary: Key studies supporting alternative diagnostic possibilities **Clinical Guidelines Documentation:** Medical guidelines supporting comprehensive evaluation approaches **Demographic-Specific Research:** Studies showing different diagnostic considerations for your population **Treatment Efficacy Research:** Evidence about expected treatment responses and timeline

Communication Record Maintenance: Keep records of all diagnostic communications:

Written Communication Copies: Emails, patient portal messages, and written requests for evaluation **Appointment Summary Documentation:** Professional summaries of verbal communications during appointments

Follow-up Request Tracking: Documentation of promised callbacks, test scheduling, and referral processing **Response Timeline Documentation:** Tracking of provider responsiveness to diagnostic concerns

When to Consider Legal Consultation

Understanding Medical Malpractice in Diagnostic Errors

Legal Standards for Diagnostic Accuracy

Diagnostic errors can constitute medical malpractice when they result from failure to meet standard of care:

Standard of Care Violations: When diagnostic approaches fall below accepted medical standards **Informed Consent Issues:** When diagnostic alternatives aren't appropriately discussed **Discrimination and Bias:** When diagnostic disparities result from inappropriate demographic assumptions **Delayed Diagnosis Harm:** When diagnostic delays result in preventable disease progression or complications

> *Legal Consultation Research Prompt: "Research the legal standards for diagnostic accuracy in [location]. What criteria indicate that diagnostic errors might warrant legal consultation, and what documentation supports malpractice claims based on misdiagnosis?"*

Exercise 8.1 – Your Diagnostic History Audit

List every diagnosis you've ever received — including the ones you now think were wrong or incomplete. Next to each one, write what symptoms were present, what tests were done, and whether the treatment actually worked.

___

___

___

___

___

___

___

___

___

___

___

___

Reflection: *Which diagnosis in your history deserves to be questioned today with what you now know?*

Exercise 8.2 – Your Alternative Diagnosis Research

Pick one diagnosis you're uncertain about. Use AI to research alternative conditions that could explain your symptom pattern. Write down at least three alternatives and what tests could help distinguish between them.

Reflection: If you could get a fresh evaluation from a provider who had never seen your chart, what would you want them to investigate?

9

STRATEGIC HEALTH COMMUNICATION BEYOND THE DOCTOR'S OFFICE

Expanding Your Healthcare Advocacy Network

Your healthcare journey extends far beyond the fifteen-minute appointment with your primary care physician. Insurance companies make coverage decisions that affect your treatment options. Healthcare administrators determine policies that influence your care access. Specialists control referral networks that can accelerate or delay your diagnosis. Hospital systems implement protocols that may work for or against your health interests.

Most patients focus their advocacy efforts solely on provider relationships, missing the broader ecosystem of healthcare decision-makers who significantly impact their health outcomes. This narrow focus leaves you vulnerable to systemic barriers, administrative denials, and institutional policies that may not serve your best interests.

This chapter will teach you to identify and influence the key decision-makers throughout the healthcare system, communicate strategically with insurance companies and administrators, build supportive networks of healthcare professionals, and create accountability systems that ensure your health interests are protected across all levels of the healthcare hierarchy.

Communicating with Insurance Companies and Healthcare Administrators

Understanding Insurance Decision-Making Frameworks

How Insurance Coverage Decisions Are Made

Insurance companies operate using complex algorithms and protocols that determine coverage for treatments, tests, and procedures. Understanding these frameworks helps you advocate more effectively:

Medical Necessity Criteria: Coverage requires demonstrated medical necessity based on established guidelines **Prior Authorization Protocols:** Many services require pre-approval based on specific clinical criteria **Step Therapy Requirements:** Insurance may require trying less expensive treatments before covering preferred options **Network Restrictions:** Coverage levels vary significantly based on provider network participation

Algorithmic Decision-Making in Insurance

Insurance companies increasingly use AI systems to make coverage decisions, which may perpetuate the same biases found in clinical AI:

Demographic Assumptions. Demographic assumptions about treatment needs can drive automated coverage decisions.
Historical Data Disparities. Historical data that reflects past healthcare disparities can perpetuate them in automated decisions.
Cost Optimization Priorities. Cost optimization algorithms may prioritize financial over health outcomes.
Automated Denial Systems. Automated denial systems often require appeals to access necessary care.

> *Insurance Algorithm Research Prompt: "Research how insurance companies use algorithms to make coverage decisions for [specific treatment/condition]. What are common reasons for denials, and what evidence is most effective in appeals for people with my profile?"*

Strategic Insurance Communication

Preparing for Insurance Interactions

Documentation Strategy for Insurance Appeals:

Medical Necessity Records. Include medical records supporting the necessity of requested treatments.
Supporting Clinical Guidelines. Reference clinical guidelines that support your treatment needs.
Demographic-Specific Research. Include research evidence for treatment effectiveness in your demographic.
Provider Justification. Attach provider recommendations with detailed medical justification.
Step Therapy Documentation. Document failed previous treatments when step therapy is required.

Language Framework for Insurance Communication

Insurance companies respond to specific types of language and evidence:

Medical Necessity Language: "This treatment is medically necessary based on [specific clinical criteria]" **Guideline Citation**: "Current [organization] guidelines recommend [treatment] for patients with [your condition and demographics]" **Evidence-Based Requests**: "Peer-reviewed research demonstrates that [treatment] is effective for [specific patient population]" **Cost-Effectiveness Arguments**: "This treatment prevents more expensive complications and reduces long-term healthcare costs"

> *Insurance Communication Prompt: "Help me draft a letter to my insurance company requesting coverage for [specific treatment]. Include medical necessity justification, relevant clinical guidelines, and evidence for effectiveness in someone with my profile: [relevant details]."*

Healthcare Administrator Advocacy

Understanding Administrative Decision-Making

Healthcare administrators operate within complex regulatory and financial frameworks:

Quality Metrics. Quality metrics that affect hospital reimbursement shape how administrators prioritize care.
Safety Protocols. Patient safety protocols that influence treatment options are shaped by institutional risk tolerance.
Efficiency Metrics. Efficiency metrics that may prioritize throughput over individualized care drive staffing and scheduling.
Regulatory Compliance. Regulatory compliance requirements shape how care is delivered and documented.

Strategic Administrative Communication

Patient Relations Departments: Use these departments strategically for communication issues **Medical Directors:** Escalate clinical care quality concerns to medical leadership **Risk Management:** Address safety concerns or potential liability issues **Quality Improvement Committees:** Participate in systematic improvement efforts

Effective Administrative Advocacy Framework:

Document Specific Issues. Provide detailed documentation of problems or concerns rather than vague complaints.
Propose Solutions. Suggest specific improvements rather than just identifying problems.
Reference Standards. Cite relevant healthcare quality standards or guidelines in your communication.
Emphasize Patient Safety. Frame issues in terms of patient safety and quality care to align with institutional priorities.
Request Written Responses. Ask for documented responses to your concerns in writing.

> *Administrative Advocacy Prompt: "Help me draft a professional communication to hospital administration about [specific issue]. Frame the concern in terms of patient safety and quality care, and propose specific solutions."*

Navigating Healthcare Systems and Bureaucracy Effectively

Healthcare System Architecture Understanding

Mapping Healthcare System Hierarchies

Clinical Hierarchy: Understanding who makes medical decisions at different levels

Attending Physicians. Attending physicians hold ultimate clinical authority for inpatient care.
Residents and NPs. Residents and nurse practitioners practice with supervised decision-making authority.
Specialists. Specialists hold expertise authority in specific areas within their domain.
Nursing Supervisors. Nursing supervisors hold care coordination authority across units and shifts.

Administrative Hierarchy: Understanding who controls policies and procedures

Department Heads. Department heads set clinical protocols for their units.
Medical Directors. Medical directors oversee quality and safety across the institution.
Hospital Administrators. Hospital administrators control resources and policies that shape patient care.
Insurance Medical Directors. Insurance medical directors make coverage decisions that affect access to care.

Information Flow Systems: Understanding how information moves through healthcare systems

EHR Systems. Electronic health record systems share clinical information across providers and settings.

Insurance Authorization. Insurance authorization systems control coverage for tests, treatments, and referrals.

Referral Systems. Referral systems connect specialists and primary care in ways that affect care coordination.

Quality Reporting. Quality reporting systems track outcomes and metrics that influence institutional priorities.

Strategic System Navigation

Leveraging System Protocols for Better Care

Patient Portal Systems: Use these strategically for communication and documentation

Permanent Written Records. Use written communication that creates permanent records.

Independent Result Access. Use test result access that allows independent analysis on your own time.

Scheduling Documentation. Use appointment scheduling that provides documentation of access issues.

Billing for Appeals. Pull billing information that supports insurance appeals.

Care Coordination Utilization: Work with care coordinators and case managers

Complex Referrals. Use care coordination for navigating complex specialty referrals.

Multi-Provider Coordination. Use care coordination for coordinating care between multiple providers.
Authorization Management. Use care coordination for managing insurance authorization requirements.
Social Services Access. Use care coordination for accessing social services and support resources.

> *System Navigation Prompt: "I'm trying to navigate [specific healthcare system challenge]. What are the most effective strategies for working within healthcare system hierarchies to achieve [specific goal]? Who are the key decision-makers I should communicate with?"*

Bureaucracy Resistance Strategies

When Standard Processes Fail

Escalation Protocols: Systematic approaches to escalating concerns

Document Initial Attempts. Record all standard process attempts and outcomes before escalating.
Identify Decision-Makers. Research who has authority to override standard processes.
Present Compelling Cases. Develop evidence-based arguments for exceptions.
Utilize External Pressure. When appropriate, involve patient advocacy organizations for outside leverage.
Legal and Regulatory Options. Understand when to involve regulatory oversight as a final escalation path.

Patient Advocacy Organization Integration

Disease-Specific Organizations: Connect with organizations focused on your specific conditions **Healthcare Access Organizations**: Utilize groups focused on healthcare equity and access **Professional Advocacy Services**: Consider professional patient advocates for complex cases **Legal Resources**: Understand when legal advocacy may be appropriate

> *Bureaucracy Navigation Prompt: "I'm facing [specific bureaucratic challenge] in accessing healthcare. What escalation strategies are most effective, and what patient advocacy resources might help with this type of issue?"*

Building Supportive Healthcare Teams and Specialist Referral Networks

Strategic Healthcare Team Development

Comprehensive Healthcare Team Architecture

Primary Care Foundation: Establishing relationships with primary care providers who understand comprehensive health advocacy **Specialist Network Development**: Building relationships with specialists who practice patient-centered care **Allied Health Integration**: Including nutritionists, mental health professionals, and other specialists **Emergency Care Planning**: Identifying emergency care providers who have access to your complete health information

Provider Vetting Strategies

Research and evaluate healthcare providers based on specific criteria:

Relevant Training and Experience. Evaluate training and experience with your specific health concerns.
Communication Approach. Assess approach to patient communication and shared decision-making.

Openness to Alternatives. Gauge willingness to consider alternative or integrative approaches.
Network Affiliations. Review network affiliations that affect referral and care coordination options.
Patient Advocacy Reviews. Look for patient reviews that indicate respect for patient concerns and advocacy.

> *Provider Research Prompt: "Help me research healthcare providers in [specialty] who demonstrate expertise in [specific condition] and patient-centered care approaches. What questions should I ask to evaluate whether a provider would be a good fit for collaborative healthcare?"*

Referral Network Optimization

Strategic Specialist Selection

Referral Timing Strategy: Understanding when specialist referrals are most beneficial

Early Specialist Referral. Seek early referral for complex or rare conditions.
Second Opinion Referral. Pursue second opinion referrals when initial evaluation is inadequate.
Preventive Specialist Consult. Consider preventive specialist consultation based on family history.
Coordinated Care Referrals. Request coordinated care referrals for multiple interrelated conditions.

Specialist Communication Coordination

Information Sharing Strategy: Ensuring all providers have necessary information

History Sharing with Specialists. Share comprehensive medical history with new specialists.
Test Result Coordination. Coordinate test results between providers to avoid duplication and confusion.
Treatment Plan Integration. Integrate treatment plans across specialties to avoid conflicts.
Communication Documentation. Document communication to prevent information loss between providers.

Multi-Specialist Care Coordination

When multiple specialists are involved in your care:

Designate Primary Coordinator. Designate a primary coordinator, often your primary care provider.
Inter-Specialist Communication. Ensure specialists communicate with each other about your care.
Prevent Conflicts. Prevent conflicting treatment recommendations by coordinating proactively.
Coordinate Appointment Timing. Coordinate appointment timing for optimal information sharing.

> *Specialist Coordination Prompt: "I'm working with multiple specialists for [condition/symptoms]. Help me develop a strategy for coordinating care between [list specialties] to ensure effective communication and integrated treatment planning."*

Using AI to Prepare for Complex Medical Discussions and Treatment Decisions

Advanced Medical Discussion Preparation

Complex Decision Analysis Framework

Use AI to help analyze complex medical decisions that involve multiple factors:

Treatment Option Analysis: Comprehensive evaluation of different treatment approaches

Demographic Effectiveness Research. Research effectiveness for your specific demographic and condition.
Side Effect Profiles. Evaluate side effect profiles and their impact on your lifestyle and health goals.
Long-Term Outcomes. Review long-term outcome research and quality of life considerations.
Alternative Options. Explore alternative treatment options that might not be initially offered.

> *Treatment Decision Analysis Prompt: "Help me analyze these treatment options for [condition]: [list options]. For someone with my profile [relevant demographics and health factors], what does research show about effectiveness, side effects, and long-term outcomes for each option?"*

Risk-Benefit Analysis for Medical Decisions

Systematic Risk Assessment: Understanding both benefits and risks of proposed treatments

Short- and Long-Term Risks. Assess short-term and long-term risk profiles of each option.

Quality of Life Impact. Conduct quality of life impact assessments for each treatment.

Alternative Risk Comparison. Compare risks across alternative options to make informed choices.

Personal Risk Tolerance. Factor in personal risk tolerance and value considerations.

Informed Consent Preparation: Going beyond basic consent forms to true understanding

Deep Procedure Research. Research procedure or treatment details beyond what providers typically discuss.

Statistical Risk Understanding. Translate statistical risk information into practical terms that inform your decision.

Informed Consent Questions. Prepare questions that ensure genuine informed consent rather than pro forma agreement.

Preference-Sensitive Decisions. Identify decision points where patient preferences significantly matter.

Shared Decision-Making Optimization

Collaborative Decision Framework Development

Value Clarification: Understanding your own priorities and preferences

Quality vs. Quantity of Life. Clarify your quality of life versus quantity of life preferences.

Outcome Risk Tolerance. Define risk tolerance levels for different types of outcomes.

Lifestyle Priorities. Identify lifestyle factor priorities that affect treatment choices.

Long-Term Goal Alignment. Ensure long-term goal alignment with treatment options.

Provider Communication Strategy for Complex Decisions

Structured Discussion Approach:

Information Gathering. Ensure you have comprehensive information about options before deciding.
Clarification Requests. Ask specific questions about unclear aspects of recommendations.
Preference Communication. Clearly express your values and priorities to guide shared decision-making.
Decision Timeline. Establish appropriate timelines for decision-making that don't rush important choices.
Follow-Up Planning. Plan ongoing communication about decision outcomes.

> *Complex Decision Communication Prompt: "I need to make a decision about [medical situation] with my healthcare provider. Help me prepare for a shared decision-making conversation that includes my values: [describe priorities] and ensures I have comprehensive information about: [specific areas of concern]."*

Creating Accountability Systems for Healthcare Providers

Systematic Provider Accountability

Performance Documentation Systems

Provider Interaction Tracking:

Communication Quality. Track communication quality and responsiveness over visits.

Clinical Decision-Making. Evaluate clinical decision-making effectiveness against outcomes.

Respect for Patient Concerns. Rate respect for patient concerns and preferences.

Follow-Through. Monitor follow-through on promises and recommendations.

Cross-Provider Coordination. Assess coordination with other providers in your care.

Outcome Measurement: Tracking healthcare effectiveness over time

Symptom Improvement. Measure symptom improvement or management success as the key outcome.

Diagnostic Accuracy. Track diagnostic accuracy and timeliness over the course of care.

Treatment Effectiveness. Evaluate treatment effectiveness and side effect management.

Overall Health Trajectory. Assess overall health trajectory under each provider's care.

> *Provider Accountability Prompt: "Help me develop a systematic approach to tracking healthcare provider performance. What metrics should I monitor to evaluate whether my providers are delivering effective, respectful care?"*

Quality Improvement Advocacy

Patient Feedback Integration

Formal Feedback Systems: Using official channels effectively

Patient Satisfaction Surveys. Complete patient satisfaction surveys strategically to influence quality improvement.

Patient Advisory Committees. Participate in patient advisory committees and councils.

Quality Improvement Participation. Join quality improvement initiatives where patient voice is valued.

Provider Evaluation Systems. Use provider evaluation systems within healthcare organizations.

Informal Accountability Networks

Peer Networks: Connecting with other patients for provider recommendations and accountability **Online Review Platforms:** Strategic use of review platforms for provider accountability **Professional Network Feedback:** Sharing experiences with healthcare professionals who can influence provider behavior **Advocacy Organization Reporting:** Reporting systemic issues to appropriate advocacy organizations

Legal and Regulatory Accountability

Understanding Patient Rights and Legal Protections

Patient Bill of Rights: Understanding specific rights within healthcare systems **Medical Malpractice Considerations:** When poor care rises to legal issues **Discrimination and Bias Reporting:** Formal channels for reporting discriminatory care **Regulatory Oversight:** When to involve state medical boards or regulatory agencies

Documentation for Accountability

Legal-Standard Documentation: Preparing documentation that could support formal complaints

Interaction and Outcome Records. Maintain detailed records of interactions and outcomes.

Dismissed Concerns Evidence. Preserve evidence of dismissed concerns or inadequate care.
Harm Documentation. Document harm resulting from poor care with specifics.
Unprofessional Behavior Communications. Keep communications that demonstrate unprofessional behavior.

> *Legal Accountability Research Prompt: "Research patient rights and legal protections in [location] for healthcare quality and discrimination issues. What documentation should I maintain, and what are the appropriate channels for reporting serious care quality concerns?"*

Technology-Enhanced Healthcare Communication

Digital Communication Optimization

Patient Portal Strategic Usage

Documentation Strategy: Using patient portals for strategic communication

Permanent Written Records. Use written communication that creates permanent records.
Pre-Appointment Question Submission. Submit questions before appointments to ensure they're addressed.
Result Review and Follow-Up. Review test results and document follow-up questions in writing.
Treatment Response Reporting. Report treatment responses for ongoing care optimization.

Telemedicine Communication Enhancement

Virtual Care Optimization: Maximizing effectiveness of remote healthcare interactions

Technical Preparation. Prepare technology to avoid communication barriers during virtual visits.
Visual Aid Sharing. Use visual aids and documentation sharing capabilities.
Virtual Follow-Up Protocols. Establish follow-up communication protocols for virtual visits.
In-Person Integration. Integrate virtual care with in-person care coordination.

> *Digital Communication Strategy Prompt: "Help me optimize my use of digital healthcare communication tools including patient portals and telemedicine platforms. What strategies ensure effective communication and documentation in digital healthcare environments?"*

AI-Enhanced Healthcare Navigation

System Navigation Support

Use AI to help navigate complex healthcare systems more effectively:

Process Optimization: Understanding efficient pathways through healthcare bureaucracy **Communication Template Development**: Creating effective templates for various healthcare communication needs **Decision Support**: Analyzing complex healthcare decisions with multiple stakeholders **Advocacy Strategy Development**: Creating systematic approaches to healthcare advocacy across different levels

> *Healthcare Navigation Prompt: "I'm navigating [specific healthcare challenge] that involves multiple stakeholders: [list stakeholders]. Help*

me develop a strategic approach that addresses each level of decision-making and maximizes my chances of achieving [specific outcome]."

Advanced Healthcare System Advocacy

Systemic Change Participation

Quality Improvement Initiative Participation

Patient Advisory Roles: Participating in healthcare system quality improvement

Hospital Patient Advisory Committees. Join hospital patient advisory committees to influence care quality.
Quality Improvement Input. Provide input on quality improvement initiatives.
Policy Consultation. Consult on policy development when invited.
Provider Training Input. Share input on provider training and education.

Research and Advocacy Integration

Patient-Centered Research: Participating in research that improves healthcare quality **Policy Advocacy**: Supporting systemic changes that improve healthcare equity **Professional Education**: Contributing to healthcare professional education about patient advocacy **Community Health Leadership**: Leading community initiatives for healthcare improvement

Healthcare Equity Advocacy

Addressing Systemic Healthcare Disparities

Bias Reporting and Documentation: Contributing to efforts to address healthcare bias **Community Health Advocacy**: Working to improve healthcare access and quality for underserved populations **Professional Training Support**: Contributing to healthcare professional bias training **Policy and Regulatory Advocacy**: Supporting regulatory changes that improve healthcare equity

> *Systemic Advocacy Planning Prompt: "Based on my healthcare experiences with [specific issues], how can I contribute to systemic improvements in healthcare quality and equity? What advocacy opportunities would be most effective given my experiences and expertise?"*

Building Comprehensive Healthcare Advocacy Networks

Strategic health communication beyond the doctor's office transforms you from an isolated patient into a connected healthcare advocate with influence across multiple levels of the healthcare system. By understanding how insurance companies, administrators, and healthcare systems operate, you can navigate bureaucracy more effectively and advocate for better care at every level.

The comprehensive approach outlined in this chapter provides frameworks for building supportive healthcare teams, creating accountability systems, and participating in systemic improvements that benefit both your individual health outcomes and broader healthcare quality. When you can communicate strategically with insurance companies, navigate healthcare bureaucracy, and build networks of supportive providers, you create a healthcare environment that works for rather than against your health interests.

Remember that healthcare advocacy is not just about individual care improvement—it's about contributing to systemic changes that improve healthcare for everyone facing similar challenges. Your experiences navigating healthcare bias, system inefficiencies, and communication barriers provide valuable insights that can inform broader healthcare improvement efforts.

Your expanded healthcare advocacy network now includes not just your clinical providers, but also administrative decision-makers, insurance advocates, and systemic change agents who can influence healthcare policy and practice. This comprehensive network provides multiple pathways for achieving better health outcomes and contributing to healthcare system improvements.

In the final chapter, we'll explore how to build your personal health intelligence network, connecting with cutting-edge research, emerging treatments, and fellow health advocates to create a comprehensive system for ongoing health optimization and advocacy development.

Exercise 9.1 – Your Support System Map

Draw a circle in the center of the page with your name in it. Around it, write the names of everyone in your health support network: family, friends, providers, patient advocates, online communities. Include contact information for each.

Reflection: *Who is missing from your network that you need to add? Who is in your network but isn't actually supportive?*

Exercise 9.2 – Your Insurance and Administrative Playbook

Write down the three most frustrating healthcare system obstacles you're currently facing (insurance denials, referral delays, test authorizations, billing disputes, etc.) and a tactical plan to address each one.

___

___

___

___

___

___

___

___

___

___

___

___

Reflection: *What's one administrative battle you've been avoiding that's affecting your care?*

10

DECODING THE HEALTHCARE HIERARCHY - UNDERSTANDING MEDICAL SPECIALTIES AND PROVIDER TYPES

Introduction: Not All Healthcare Providers Are Created Equal

When you schedule an appointment for chest pain, the difference between seeing a family medicine physician, a physician assistant, or a cardiologist could literally be the difference between life and death. Yet most patients remain unaware of the vast differences in training, expertise, and scope of practice among healthcare providers. This knowledge gap leaves you vulnerable to receiving care from providers whose training may not match your health needs, missing opportunities for specialized expertise, or accepting limitations that don't actually exist.

The healthcare hierarchy is complex and intentionally opaque. Hospitals and clinics often present all providers as equivalent, using terms like "provider" or "clinician" that obscure important differences in education, training, and capability. Understanding these distinctions empowers you to make informed decisions about who provides your care, when to insist on specific provider types, and how to navigate the system to access the expertise you need.

This chapter will decode the healthcare hierarchy systematically, explaining the education and training differences among provider types, the scope and limitations of each role, and strategic approaches to selecting providers whose expertise matches your health needs. You'll learn to research provider credentials effectively, understand the 24 primary medical specialties and their subspecialties, and navigate referral systems to access specialized care when standard primary care approaches prove inadequate.

Understanding Healthcare Provider Education and Training Hierarchies

Medical Doctors (MD and DO): The Foundation of Medical Practice

Doctor of Medicine (MD) Education and Training

Medical doctors represent the most extensively trained healthcare providers, with education specifically designed to diagnose and treat the full spectrum of human disease:

Undergraduate Education (4 years): Bachelor's degree with prerequisite courses in sciences, though any major is acceptable **Medical College Admission Test (MCAT):** Standardized exam testing knowledge in biological sciences, physical sciences, and critical thinking

Medical School (4 years): Two years of basic science education followed by two years of clinical rotations across all major specialties **United States Medical Licensing Examination (USMLE)**: Three-part examination sequence testing medical knowledge and clinical skills **Residency Training (3-7 years)**: Intensive supervised clinical training in chosen specialty with progressively increasing responsibility **Board Certification**: Examination by specialty board confirming expertise in chosen field **Optional Fellowship Training (1-3 years)**: Subspecialty training for highly specialized areas of medicine

Doctor of Osteopathic Medicine (DO) Education and Training

DOs receive equivalent medical training with additional emphasis on musculoskeletal system and osteopathic manipulative treatment:

Equivalent Academic Requirements: Same undergraduate prerequisites and medical school duration as MD programs **Osteopathic Principles Integration**: Additional training in whole-person approach and osteopathic manipulative medicine **Residency and Fellowship**: Can complete training in MD or DO programs, with identical requirements for board certification **Scope of Practice**: Identical to MDs in all states, with ability to prescribe medications, perform surgery, and practice in all medical specialties

> *MD vs DO Research Prompt: "Research the practical differences between MD and DO training for [specific specialty]. What osteopathic approaches might benefit someone with my health conditions [describe conditions]?"*

Physician Assistants (PAs): Mid-Level Providers with Supervision Requirements

Physician Assistant Education and Training

PAs receive accelerated medical training designed to provide healthcare under physician supervision:

Prerequisite Education: Bachelor's degree preferred, though some programs accept less, typically with healthcare experience requirements **PA Program Duration:** 24-32 months of intensive didactic and clinical training **Clinical Rotations:** Shorter rotations across major medical specialties, typically 4-8 weeks each compared to 6-12 weeks for medical students **Certification Examination:** National certification exam administered by National Commission on Certification of Physician Assistants **Continuing Education:** 100 hours every two years plus certification maintenance exam every ten years **Supervision Requirements:** Must practice under physician supervision, though degree of supervision varies by state

PA Scope of Practice and Limitations

Diagnostic Authority: Can diagnose conditions within their training and experience, but complex or unusual cases should be referred **Prescriptive Authority:** Can prescribe medications, including controlled substances in most states, under physician supervision **Procedural Capabilities:** Can perform procedures within their training, though complex procedures typically require physician oversight **Independent Practice Limitations:** Cannot practice independently; must maintain supervisory relationship with physician

> *PA Scope Research Prompt: "Research PA scope of practice in [state] for [specific condition/procedure]. What are the supervision requirements, and when should I request physician evaluation instead of PA care?"*

Nurse Practitioners (NPs): Advanced Practice Nursing with Variable Training

Nurse Practitioner Education and Training Pathways

NP training varies significantly based on program type and specialty focus:

RN License Requirement: Must first obtain registered nurse license and typically some clinical nursing experience **Graduate Education**: Master's degree (minimum) or Doctor of Nursing Practice (DNP), though requirements vary significantly **Specialty Focus**: Training focused on specific populations (family, adult, pediatric, psychiatric, etc.) rather than broad medical education **Clinical Hours**: Requirements vary dramatically between programs, from 500 to 1,500+ hours **Certification**: National certification in chosen specialty area **Independent Practice**: Varies by state from full practice authority to physician supervision requirements

NP Training Variability and Quality Concerns

Program Inconsistency: Significant variation in admission requirements, clinical training, and academic rigor between programs **Online Programs**: Many NP programs offer online formats with limited clinical oversight **Experience Requirements**: Some programs accept nurses with minimal bedside experience **Specialty Limitations**: Training focused on specific populations may limit ability to recognize conditions outside specialty area

Direct-Entry Programs: Some programs accept candidates without nursing experience, providing accelerated pathway to NP certification

> *NP Quality Research Prompt: "Research NP training programs in [area] for [specialty]. What program characteristics indicate rigorous training, and how can I evaluate whether a specific NP received comprehensive education?"*

Familiar Medical Specialties: Understanding Expertise Areas and Applications

Primary Care Specialties: The Foundation of Healthcare

Family Medicine

Family medicine physicians provide comprehensive healthcare across all ages and conditions:

Training Focus: Three-year residency covering internal medicine, pediatrics, obstetrics/gynecology, surgery, and psychiatry **Scope of Practice**: Preventive care, chronic disease management, acute illness treatment, basic procedures **Appropriate Uses**: Routine healthcare, health maintenance, uncomplicated chronic conditions, coordination of specialist care **Limitations**: Complex conditions requiring specialized diagnostic or treatment approaches

Internal Medicine

Internists specialize in adult medicine with focus on diagnosis and non-surgical treatment:

Training Focus: Three-year residency in adult medicine, with emphasis on complex medical conditions **Scope of Practice**: Adult preventive care, complex medical conditions, diagnostic evaluation, chronic disease management **Subspecialty Options**: Cardiology, gastroenterology, endocrinology, and 17 other subspecialties **Appropriate Uses**: Complex adult medical conditions, diagnostic challenges, multiple chronic conditions

Obstetrics and Gynecology (OB/GYN)

OB/GYNs specialize in the female reproductive system and the management of pregnancy and childbirth:

Training Focus: Four-year residency combining medical and surgical training in female reproductive health, pregnancy, and hormones.

Scope of Practice: Reproductive health, prenatal and postpartum care, hormone management (menopause/PCOS), and surgical procedures (hysterectomies, fibroid removal).

Unique Role: For many women, the OB/GYN serves as a **primary care provider**, often being the first to identify systemic issues like thyroid dysfunction or autoimmune markers.

Appropriate Uses: Annual screenings, pregnancy management, pelvic pain, hormonal imbalances, and reproductive system surgeries.

Limitations: While they handle hormonal health, complex systemic metabolic issues may still require a co-managed approach with an **Endocrinologist**.

Pediatrics

Pediatricians specialize in healthcare for infants, children, and adolescents:

Training Focus: Three-year residency in child and adolescent medicine and development **Age Range**: Birth through age 18 (sometimes extended to age 21) **Subspecialty Options**: Pediatric subspecialties parallel adult medicine (pediatric cardiology, pediatric endocrinology, etc.) **Appropriate Uses**: All healthcare needs for children and adolescents

> *Primary Care Selection Prompt: "Based on my age [age], health conditions [list conditions], and healthcare needs [describe needs], which primary care specialty would be most appropriate? What questions should I ask when evaluating primary care providers?"*

General Surgery

General surgeons perform operations on abdomen, breast, skin, soft tissues, and other areas:

Training Duration: Five-year residency following medical school **Common Procedures:** Appendectomy, gallbladder surgery, hernia repair, breast surgery, skin cancer removal **Subspecialty Options:** Trauma surgery, critical care surgery, breast surgery, others **Appropriate Uses:** Surgical conditions within general surgery scope

Orthopedic Surgery

Orthopedic surgeons treat musculoskeletal system conditions:

Training Focus: Five-year residency in bones, joints, muscles, ligaments, and tendons **Common Procedures:** Joint replacement, fracture repair, arthroscopy, spine surgery **Subspecialties:** Sports medicine, spine surgery, hand surgery, joint replacement **Appropriate Uses:** Bone fractures, joint problems, sports injuries, spine conditions

Neurosurgery

Neurosurgeons perform surgery on brain, spine, and nervous system:

Training Duration: Seven-year residency (longest surgical training) **Scope:** Brain tumors, aneurysms, spine conditions, traumatic brain injury **Highly Specialized:** Most complex surgical specialty with extensive subspecialization **Appropriate Uses:** Brain and spinal cord conditions requiring surgical intervention

Cardiology

Cardiologists specialize in heart and cardiovascular system:

Training: Three-year internal medicine residency plus three-year cardiology fellowship **Scope:** Heart disease diagnosis, treatment, and prevention **Subspecialties:** Interventional cardiology, electrophysiology, heart failure, others **Appropriate Uses:** Heart conditions, chest pain evaluation, cardiovascular risk assessment

Endocrinology

Endocrinologists treat hormone-related conditions:

Training: Internal medicine residency plus two-year endocrinology fellowship **Common Conditions:** Diabetes, thyroid disorders, adrenal conditions, reproductive hormone issues **Appropriate Uses:** Complex hormone problems, diabetes management, unexplained metabolic symptoms

Gastroenterology

Gastroenterologists treat digestive system conditions:

Training: Internal medicine residency plus three-year gastroenterology fellowship **Procedures:** Endoscopy, colonoscopy, liver biopsy **Appropriate Uses:** Digestive problems, abdominal pain, inflammatory bowel disease

> *Specialty Selection Research Prompt: "Based on my symptoms [describe symptoms] and failed treatments [list treatments], which medical specialty would be most appropriate for evaluation? What questions should I ask when requesting specialist referral?"*

Oncology

Oncologists specialize in the diagnosis and treatment of cancer. Because cancer care is complex, your readers will likely encounter a **multidisciplinary team.**

Training Focus: Internal medicine residency followed by a fellowship in medical oncology.

Three Main Sub-Specialties:

Medical Oncologist. The "quarterback" of the team who uses systemic treatments like chemotherapy, immunotherapy, and targeted therapies that work throughout the body.
Surgical Oncologist. Specializes in the physical removal of tumors and performing biopsies.
Radiation Oncologist. Uses high-energy X-rays or particles to target and destroy cancer cells in a specific location.
Appropriate Uses. Unexplained weight loss, persistent lumps, abnormal imaging (found by a Radiologist), or a confirmed cancer diagnosis.
Limitations. They focus on the cancer itself; for systemic hormone issues caused by treatment, a patient may still need an Endocrinologist.

Urology

Urologists treat conditions of the **urinary tract**(kidneys, bladder, ureters, and urethra) in both men and women, as well as the male reproductive system.

Training Focus. A five- to six-year surgical residency focusing on both medical and surgical management of the urinary system.
Appropriate Uses for Women. Chronic UTIs, urinary incontinence, kidney stones, bladder pain (interstitial cystitis), and pelvic floor dysfunction.
Common Misconception. Many women believe urinary issues are only for their OB/GYN, but a Urologist has more specialized surgical and diagnostic tools for the bladder and kidneys.
Subspecialty Note. A Urologic Oncologist is a surgeon who specifically treats cancers of the urinary system, such as bladder or kidney cancer.

Diagnostic Specialties: Behind-the-Scenes Expertise

Radiology

Radiologists interpret medical imaging studies:

Training: Four-year residency plus optional fellowship training **Subspecialties**: Neuroradiology, interventional radiology, breast imaging, others **Direct Patient Contact**: Usually limited, though interventional radiologists perform procedures **Importance**: Critical for accurate diagnosis through imaging interpretation

Pathology

Pathologists diagnose disease through laboratory analysis:

Training: Four-year residency in anatomic pathology, clinical pathology, or both **Scope**: Tissue biopsy interpretation, blood test analysis, autopsy examination **Patient Contact**: Rarely direct, but crucial for accurate diagnosis **Subspecialties**: Surgical pathology, hematopathology, forensic pathology

Nuclear Medicine

Nuclear medicine physicians use radioactive materials for diagnosis and treatment:

Training: Four-year residency in nuclear medicine **Procedures**: PET scans, bone scans, cardiac stress tests, thyroid treatments **Appropriate Uses**: Specialized imaging needs, certain cancer treatments

Strategic Provider Selection and Credential Research

Evaluating Provider Credentials and Experience

Board Certification Verification

Board certification represents completion of specialized training and examination:

Verification Resources: American Board of Medical Specialties (ABMS) website for MDs/DOs, specialty organization websites for other providers **Certification Maintenance**: Most specialties require ongoing education and periodic re-certification **Subspecialty Certification**: Additional training and certification in narrower expertise areas

> *Board Certification Research Prompt: "Verify the board certification status for [provider name] and research what their specific certifications mean for treating conditions like mine [describe conditions]."*

Training Institution and Program Quality

Residency and fellowship training quality varies significantly between institutions:

Academic Medical Centers: University hospitals typically provide more comprehensive training **Program Reputation**: Some training programs have better reputations for producing excellent physicians **Training Volume**: Programs with higher patient volumes typically provide more experience **Fellowship Training**: Additional subspecialty training indicates higher expertise in specific areas

Clinical Experience and Patient Population

Years in Practice: Experience level appropriate for your condition complexity **Patient Demographics**: Experience treating patients similar to you in age, gender, ethnicity **Condition-Specific Experience**: Volume of patients with your specific condition **Outcome Data**: When available, success rates for procedures or treatments

> *Provider Experience Research Prompt: "Research [provider name]'s training background and experience treating [specific condition] in patients with my demographics [age, gender, relevant factors]. What questions should I ask about their experience with cases like mine?"*

Hospital Affiliation and System Quality Research

Hospital Quality Metrics and Rankings

Hospital affiliations affect provider capabilities and resource access:

Quality Ratings: Leapfrog Group, Healthgrades, and US News rankings **Specialty Recognition**: Centers of excellence designations for specific conditions **Academic Affiliations**: Teaching hospitals often have access to latest treatments and research **Technology Access**: Advanced diagnostic and treatment capabilities

System Resources and Coordination

Multidisciplinary Care: Ability to coordinate care among multiple specialists **Research Access**: Participation in clinical trials and access to experimental treatments **Emergency Capabilities**: Trauma center level and emergency service capabilities **Insurance Relationships**: Network participation and coverage considerations

Geographic and Access Considerations

Travel Distance vs. Expertise Trade-offs

Sometimes the best expertise requires traveling beyond your immediate area:

Local Capability Assessment: Evaluate whether local providers have adequate expertise for your needs **Regional Medical Centers:** Major cities typically have more specialized expertise **Travel Feasibility:** Consider travel requirements for ongoing care versus one-time consultation **Telemedicine Options:** Some specialists offer remote consultation or follow-up care

> *Geographic Access Research Prompt: "Compare local provider options for [condition] with regional medical centers within [distance] miles. What level of expertise is available locally versus what I might access by traveling?"*

Understanding Referral Networks and Insurance Navigation

Referral System Mechanics and Strategy

Primary Care Referral Requirements

Most insurance plans require primary care referrals for specialist access:

Referral Timing: How quickly referrals get processed and appointments scheduled **Referral Specifications:** Whether referrals specify particular specialists or allow patient choice **Authorization Requirements:** Additional insurance authorizations needed for certain specialists **Network Limitations:** Referrals typically limited to in-network providers

Strategic Referral Advocacy

Specific Specialist Requests: Research and request referral to specific providers rather than accepting generic referrals **Urgent Referral Justification:** When symptoms warrant expedited specialist evaluation **Out-of-Network Referral Advocacy:** Building cases for accessing out-of-network expertise when necessary **Multiple Referral Requests:** When complex conditions require evaluation by multiple specialists

> *Referral Strategy Prompt: "I need referral to [specific specialist type] for [condition/symptoms]. Help me prepare a request to my primary care provider that justifies referral to a specific specialist and expedited evaluation."*

Insurance Authorization and Prior Authorization Navigation

Prior Authorization Requirements and Strategy

Many specialists and procedures require insurance pre-approval:

Pre-Authorization Research: Understanding which services require prior authorization **Medical Necessity Documentation:** Building cases that demonstrate medical necessity for coverage **Appeal Processes:** When initial authorizations are denied **Timeline Management:** Planning around authorization processing times

Coverage Optimization Strategies

Network Provider Research: Finding high-quality providers within insurance networks **Out-of-Network Benefits:** Understanding when out-of-network providers might be covered **Appeal Rights:** Insurance appeal processes for denied coverage **Financial Assistance:** Hospital and provider financial assistance programs

Building Long-Term Specialist Relationships

Multi-Specialty Care Coordination

For complex conditions requiring multiple specialists:

Care Coordination: Ensuring specialists communicate effectively with each other **Primary Coordinator:** Designating a primary provider to coordinate overall care **Information Sharing:** Ensuring all providers have access to complete medical records **Treatment Plan Integration:** Avoiding conflicting recommendations from different specialists

Specialist Relationship Maintenance

Regular Communication: Staying in touch with specialists for ongoing conditions **Preventive Consultation:** Consulting specialists preventively based on family history or risk factors **Second Opinion Relationships:** Maintaining relationships with alternative specialists for complex decisions **Emergency Access:** Understanding how to access specialist care in urgent situations

> *Multi-Specialist Coordination Prompt: "I'm working with specialists in [list specialties] for [condition/symptoms]. Help me develop a strategy for ensuring effective coordination and communication among my healthcare team."*

Advanced Provider Selection Strategies

Academic vs. Community Practice Considerations

Academic Medical Centers

University hospitals and academic medical centers offer unique advantages:

Research Access: Participation in clinical trials and access to experimental treatments **Subspecialty Expertise:** Highly specialized providers who focus on narrow areas of expertise **Multidisciplinary Clinics:** Team-based approaches to complex conditions **Teaching Environment:** Providers stay current with latest research and developments

Potential Limitations: Longer wait times, less continuity, trainee involvement in care

Community Practice Advantages

Private practice and community providers may offer:

Accessibility: Shorter wait times and more flexible scheduling **Continuity:** Long-term relationships with consistent providers **Efficiency:** Streamlined care without academic obligations **Local Convenience:** Proximity to home and integrated with local healthcare systems

> *Academic vs Community Research Prompt: "Compare academic medical center options with community providers in [area] for [specific condition]. What are the trade-offs in expertise, accessibility, and care coordination for someone with my needs?"*

Provider Communication Style and Philosophy Assessment

Patient-Centered Care Evaluation

Shared Decision-Making: Providers who involve patients in treatment decisions **Communication Quality:** Clear explanation of conditions, treatments, and alternatives **Cultural Competence:** Understanding and respect for diverse patient backgrounds **Bias Awareness:** Recognition and active efforts to address healthcare disparities

Evaluation Strategies

Initial Consultation Assessment: Using first appointments to evaluate provider approach **Question Response Quality:** How providers respond to patient questions and concerns **Research Discussion:** Willingness to discuss patient research and alternative approaches **Advocacy Support:** Support for patient self-advocacy and second opinion seeking

> *Provider Philosophy Assessment Prompt: "Prepare interview questions to evaluate whether a potential provider practices patient-centered care and would be supportive of my healthcare advocacy approach. What indicators suggest a provider would work collaboratively with informed patients?"*

Specialized and Concierge Care Options

Direct Primary Care and Concierge Medicine

Alternative payment models that may provide enhanced access:

Direct Primary Care: Monthly membership fee for enhanced primary care access **Concierge Medicine:** Enhanced primary care with more time, access, and coordination **Benefits:** Longer appointments, better accessibility, enhanced coordination **Limitations:** Additional costs, potential limitations in specialist integration

Specialized Medical Centers

Centers focused on specific conditions or approaches:

Disease-Specific Centers: Facilities specializing in particular conditions (cancer centers, heart institutes) **Integrative Medicine Centers:** Facilities combining conventional and complementary approaches **Women's Health Centers:** Specialized focus on conditions affecting women **Diagnostic Centers:** Facilities specializing in complex diagnostic evaluation

Specialized Care Research Prompt: "Research specialized medical centers for [specific condition] that might provide more comprehensive care than traditional healthcare settings. What advantages might these centers offer for someone with my health profile?"

Technology Integration and Telemedicine Considerations

Digital Health Platform Evaluation

Telemedicine Quality Assessment

Provider Qualifications: Ensuring remote providers meet same standards as in-person care **Technology Platforms:** Evaluating security, functionality, and integration capabilities **Appropriate Use Cases:** Understanding when telemedicine is appropriate versus when in-person evaluation is necessary **Integration with Local Care:** How telemedicine providers coordinate with local healthcare teams

Digital Health Records and Coordination

Health Information Exchange: How different providers and systems share information **Patient Portal Functionality:** Tools for communication, appointment scheduling, and record access **Wearable Device Integration:** Providers who utilize health monitoring technology data **AI-Enhanced Care:** Providers using artificial intelligence tools to enhance diagnostic and treatment capabilities

Future Healthcare Delivery Models

Emerging Care Models

Virtual-First Primary Care: Primary care delivered primarily through digital platforms **AI-Augmented Diagnosis**: Providers using artificial intelligence to enhance diagnostic accuracy **Precision Medicine Integration**: Providers incorporating genetic and biomarker testing into treatment planning **Value-Based Care**: Payment models focused on health outcomes rather than service volume

> *Future Care Model Research Prompt: "Research emerging healthcare delivery models in [area] that might provide more personalized, technology-enhanced care for someone with my health profile [describe relevant factors]."*

Conclusion: Mastering Healthcare Navigation Through Provider Intelligence

Understanding the healthcare hierarchy transforms you from a passive recipient of assigned care into an informed consumer who can select providers whose expertise, training, and approach match your health needs. The systematic approach to provider evaluation outlined in this chapter ensures that you work with providers who have appropriate training for your conditions, experience with your demographic, and commitment to patient-centered care.

The distinctions between provider types—from the extensive training of medical doctors to the focused expertise of specialists to the supervised practice of mid-level providers—directly impact the quality and appropriateness of your care. When you understand these differences, you can advocate for provider types whose scope of practice matches your healthcare needs and request specialist referrals when conditions exceed primary care capabilities.

Your ability to research provider credentials, evaluate training backgrounds, and assess hospital affiliations empowers you to make informed decisions about where to seek care and which providers to trust with your health. This knowledge becomes particularly important when dealing with complex conditions, seeking second opinions, or navigating emergency situations where provider selection can significantly impact outcomes.

The healthcare system's complexity and opacity work against patients who don't understand provider hierarchies and referral systems. By mastering this knowledge, you gain the ability to navigate efficiently toward appropriate expertise, avoid delays caused by inadequate provider selection, and build healthcare teams whose combined expertise addresses your complete health profile.

Remember that the healthcare hierarchy exists to organize expertise appropriately—when you understand this organization, you can leverage it to your advantage rather than being constrained by artificial barriers or inadequate provider assignments. Your health deserves care from providers whose training and expertise match your needs, and this chapter provides the tools to ensure that match occurs consistently.

Your provider selection and healthcare navigation skills become the foundation for all other advocacy efforts outlined in this book. When you work with appropriate providers who respect patient advocacy and practice evidence-based medicine, every other aspect of healthcare advocacy—from diagnostic accuracy to treatment optimization—becomes more achievable and effective.

In the next chapter, we'll build on this provider knowledge to explore routine lab work interpretation, ensuring you understand not just who should order and interpret your tests, but what those results actually mean for your health optimization and disease prevention efforts.

Exercise 10.1 – Your Specialist Needs Assessment

List every specialist you think you need to see and WHY. Then rank them by urgency. Next to each, write whether you currently have a referral and what's standing in the way of making the appointment.

____

____

____

____

____

____

____

____

____

____

____

____

Reflection: *Which specialist have you been putting off because you're afraid of what they might find?*

Exercise 10.2 – Your Provider Evaluation Criteria

Write down the qualities you want in your ideal healthcare provider. Be specific: communication style, willingness to collaborate, openness to patient research, demographic awareness, etc. Use this list when evaluating new providers.

Reflection: *How many of your current providers actually meet these criteria? Which ones should you replace?*

11

BUILDING YOUR PERSONAL HEALTH INTELLIGENCE NETWORK

Beyond Individual Advocacy to Collective Intelligence

The healthcare advocacy skills you've developed throughout this book transform you from a passive patient into an informed health advocate. However, individual advocacy, while powerful, has limitations. The most sophisticated health advocates understand that sustainable healthcare transformation requires building networks of intelligence, support, and collective action that extend far beyond individual provider relationships.

Your personal health intelligence network encompasses the research resources, professional relationships, peer connections, and technological tools that support ongoing health optimization and advocacy development. This network provides access to cutting-edge research before it reaches mainstream medical practice, connects you with fellow advocates facing similar challenges, and creates pathways for contributing to healthcare system improvements that benefit broader communities.

Building this network isn't about replacing medical professionals or creating echo chambers that reinforce confirmation bias. Instead, it's about creating a sophisticated information ecosystem that helps you stay current with health innovations, validates your advocacy approaches, and provides support for navigating complex healthcare challenges.

This chapter will teach you to identify and connect with cutting-edge health research, build relationships with healthcare professionals who value patient partnership, create supportive peer networks, and establish systems for ongoing health advocacy development that benefit both your individual health and broader healthcare equity efforts.

Connecting with Other Patients and Health Advocates Using AI Research Tools

Strategic Peer Network Development

Identifying High-Quality Patient Communities

Not all patient communities provide reliable health information or effective advocacy support. Use AI to help evaluate and connect with communities that maintain high standards for information sharing and mutual support:

> *Community Evaluation Prompt: "Research patient communities and advocacy groups for [specific condition/demographic]. What organizations maintain evidence-based approaches to health information sharing and demonstrate effective advocacy outcomes? What criteria should I use to evaluate patient community quality?"*

Building Meaningful Peer Connections

Shared Experience Networks: Connect with people facing similar health challenges or advocacy experiences **Demographic-Specific Groups:** Communities focused on health issues affecting your specific demographic **Geographic Communities:** Local networks that understand regional healthcare system challenges **Professional Networks:** Connections with healthcare professionals who support patient advocacy

AI-Enhanced Community Engagement

Research-Driven Community Participation

Use AI to enhance your contributions to patient communities:

> *Community Contribution Strategy: "I want to contribute meaningfully to [specific patient community]. Based on my experiences with [health challenges/advocacy successes], how can I share information that helps others while maintaining appropriate boundaries about medical advice?"*

Collaborative Research Projects

Many patient communities engage in collaborative research that can benefit broader understanding of health conditions:

Patient-Reported Outcome Studies. Participate in patient-reported outcome studies that measure real-world experience.
Treatment Effectiveness Surveys. Contribute to treatment effectiveness surveys that capture patient perspective.
Healthcare Quality Assessment. Join healthcare quality assessment projects to improve care delivery.
Advocacy Strategy Sharing. Document and share advocacy strategies that work for others.

Information Validation Networks

Develop systems for validating health information through peer networks:

Cross-Reference with Advocates. Cross-reference research findings with other advocates to confirm accuracy.
Share Provider Experiences. Share provider recommendations and experiences across networks.
Collaborative Evaluation. Evaluate new treatments or research collaboratively with other informed patients.
Group System Analysis. Conduct group analysis of healthcare system challenges and solutions.

Finding Cutting-Edge Research and Clinical Trials Relevant to Your Conditions

Advanced Medical Research Navigation

Beyond Standard Literature Searches

Most patients limit their research to basic Google searches or mainstream health websites. Sophisticated health advocates access the same research resources used by healthcare professionals:

Primary Research Sources:

PubMed. Use PubMed for peer-reviewed medical literature searches.
ClinicalTrials.gov. Use ClinicalTrials.gov for current and upcoming research studies.
Cochrane Reviews. Use Cochrane Reviews for systematic analysis of treatment effectiveness.

Professional Guidelines. Consult professional medical organization guidelines and position statements.

Advanced Research Strategy Prompt: "Help me develop a systematic approach to staying current with research on [specific conditions/interests]. What databases, search strategies, and alert systems will help me access cutting-edge research before it reaches mainstream medical practice?"

Clinical Trial Identification and Evaluation

Trial Participation Consideration: Research clinical trials that might be appropriate for your health profile:

New Treatment Trials. Consider trials investigating new treatments for your conditions.
Prevention Studies. Consider prevention studies for conditions in your family history.
Quality of Life Research. Consider quality of life or symptom management research.
Diagnostic Accuracy Studies. Consider diagnostic accuracy or early detection studies.

Trial Evaluation Criteria:

Relevance to Your Goals. Evaluate research question relevance to your health goals.
Study Design and Safety. Review study design quality and safety protocols.
Investigator Credentials. Check investigator credentials and institutional reputation.
Benefit–Risk Assessment. Assess potential benefits versus risks for your specific situation.

Clinical Trial Research Prompt: "Based on my health profile [relevant details], research current clinical trials that might be appropriate for someone with my conditions and demographics. What trials are investigating [specific treatments/approaches], and what criteria should I use to evaluate trial participation?"

Emerging Treatment and Technology Monitoring

Innovation Pipeline Tracking

Stay informed about health innovations before they become widely available:

Emerging Diagnostics. Track emerging diagnostic technologies relevant to your conditions.
New Treatments in Development. Follow new treatment approaches in development.
Medical Device Innovations. Monitor medical device innovations that may benefit you.
Digital Health Tools. Watch digital health tool development that supports your advocacy.

International Research Integration

Healthcare innovations often emerge in different countries before reaching your healthcare system:

European Research. European research may lead future treatment approaches that eventually reach US care.
Asian Medical Innovations. Asian medical innovations, particularly in integrative medicine, offer alternative models.
Canadian Healthcare Innovations. Canadian healthcare system innovations focus on access and equity.
Developing Country Innovations. Developing country innovations in cost-effective healthcare delivery can inform resource-limited advocacy.

Global Research Monitoring Prompt: "Help me identify international research and healthcare innovations relevant to [specific health interests]. What countries or research institutions are leading innovation in these areas, and how can I stay informed about developments that may eventually reach my healthcare system?"

Using AI to Track Health Trends and Emerging Treatment Options

Systematic Trend Analysis

Health Trend Identification Systems

Use AI to identify and analyze health trends that might affect your care:

Trend Analysis Setup: "Help me create a system for monitoring health trends related to [specific conditions/demographics]. What indicators suggest emerging treatment options, changing diagnostic approaches, or evolving understanding of my health conditions?"

Treatment Evolution Tracking

Monitor how treatment approaches evolve over time:

Standard of Care Changes. Track standard of care changes in your conditions over time.
Alternative Treatment Evidence. Monitor emerging evidence for alternative treatment approaches.
Technology in Treatment Delivery. Watch for technology integration in treatment delivery.
Personalized Medicine. Follow personalized medicine developments relevant to your conditions.

Predictive Health Intelligence

Personal Health Forecasting

Use trend analysis to anticipate future health needs and opportunities:

Upcoming Treatment Options. Anticipate treatment options likely to become available in your timeframe.
Emerging Diagnostic Monitoring. Identify diagnostic technologies that might benefit your health monitoring.
Research-Backed Prevention. Track prevention strategies gaining research support.
Delivery Innovations. Note healthcare delivery innovations that might improve access.

Risk and Opportunity Assessment

> *Future Planning Analysis: "Based on current research trends and my health profile [relevant details], what health innovations or treatment developments should I monitor for potential benefit? What timeline considerations should guide my health planning and advocacy efforts?"*

Building Relationships with Healthcare Professionals Who Value Patient Partnership

Identifying Partnership-Oriented Providers

Professional Advocacy Network Development

Research-Active Providers: Healthcare professionals engaged in research who understand evolving medical knowledge **Equity-Focused Practitioners:** Providers who demonstrate commitment to addressing healthcare disparities **Integrative Approach Providers:** Professionals who value collaboration with patients and other healthcare approaches **Educational Institution Affiliations:** Providers connected to teaching institutions who value shared learning

Provider Partnership Evaluation

Assess healthcare providers for genuine partnership orientation:

Research Discussion Willingness. Assess willingness to discuss current research and emerging treatments.
Respect for Patient Advocacy. Evaluate respect for patient research and advocacy efforts.
Collaborative Approach. Look for a collaborative approach to treatment planning and decision-making.
Support for Referrals. Seek providers who support patient connections with appropriate specialists or resources.

> *Provider Partnership Assessment: "Help me develop criteria for evaluating whether healthcare providers genuinely support patient partnership and advocacy. What questions and observations will help me identify providers who value collaborative healthcare relationships?"*

Professional Relationship Development

Long-Term Partnership Building

Educational Exchange: Share relevant research and advocacy experiences with providers who demonstrate openness **Collaborative Learning:** Participate in provider education about patient experiences and perspectives **Professional Development Support:** Support provider efforts to improve healthcare equity and patient advocacy **Referral Network Integration:** Connect with providers who maintain networks of partnership-oriented colleagues

Mutual Professional Respect

Develop relationships based on mutual expertise recognition:

Acknowledge Expertise Both Ways. Acknowledge provider clinical expertise while asserting patient expertise about personal health experiences.
Share Advocacy Insights. Share research and advocacy insights that might benefit provider practice.
Provide Feedback. Provide feedback about care quality and communication effectiveness.
Support Provider Equity Efforts. Support provider efforts to improve healthcare access and equity.

Creating Long-Term Health Optimization and Prevention Strategies

Comprehensive Life-Stage Health Planning

Predictive Health Strategy Development

Use family history intelligence, current research, and personal health data to develop comprehensive prevention strategies:

> *Life-Stage Planning Analysis: "Based on my family health patterns [relevant history], current health data [relevant information], and research on prevention for my demographic, help me develop long-term health optimization strategies for different life stages. What prevention approaches show strongest evidence for people with my risk profile?"*

Adaptive Strategy Framework

Develop health strategies that evolve with new research and changing health needs:

Regular Strategy Review. Review and update strategy regularly based on new research.
Flexibility to Incorporate New Approaches. Remain flexible to incorporate emerging prevention or treatment approaches.
Technology Integration. Integrate new health technologies and monitoring tools as they become available.
Life-Stage Adaptation. Adapt to changing life circumstances and health priorities over time.

Technology Integration for Health Optimization

Digital Health Tool Integration

Wearable Technology: Strategic use of health monitoring devices for ongoing optimization **AI Health Analysis:** Platforms that provide personalized health insights based on individual data **Telemedicine Integration:** Remote healthcare access that supports ongoing monitoring and optimization **Health Record Management:** Digital systems for comprehensive health information management

Future Technology Preparation

Prepare for emerging health technologies that may benefit your optimization efforts:

Genetic Testing. Prepare for genetic testing and analysis for personalized medicine.
Advanced Biomarkers. Consider advanced biomarker testing for early detection and optimization.
AI Diagnostic Tools. Watch AI-powered diagnostic tools that may improve healthcare accuracy.
Personalized Medicine Approaches. Pursue personalized medicine approaches based on individual health profiles.

Technology Integration Planning: "Help me develop a strategic approach to integrating current and emerging health technologies into my health optimization efforts. What technologies show strongest evidence for people with my health profile, and how should I evaluate new health technology offerings?"

Advanced Network Development and Maintenance

Strategic Network Architecture

Multi-Level Network Design

Individual Level: Personal relationships with healthcare providers, advocates, and peers **Organizational Level:** Connections with advocacy organizations, research institutions, and healthcare systems **Community Level:** Local networks focused on healthcare access and quality improvement **Professional Level:** Relationships with healthcare professionals who support patient advocacy

Network Maintenance and Development

Regular Communication: Systematic approaches to maintaining valuable network relationships **Mutual Support:** Contributing to network members' advocacy and health goals **Information Sharing:** Strategic sharing of research, resources, and advocacy insights **Collaborative Projects:** Participating in group efforts that benefit network members and broader communities

Knowledge Sharing and Community Leadership

Expertise Development and Sharing

Transform your advocacy experience into expertise that benefits others:

Document Successful Strategies. Document successful advocacy strategies and approaches to share with others.
Share Research and Navigation. Share research insights and healthcare navigation experiences.
Mentor New Advocates. Mentor other patients beginning advocacy journeys.
Contribute to Training. Contribute to patient education and advocacy training programs.

Community Health Leadership

Local Leadership: Lead community efforts to improve healthcare access and quality **Professional Collaboration**: Work with healthcare professionals to improve patient advocacy support **Policy Advocacy**: Support legislative and regulatory changes that improve healthcare equity **Educational Contributions**: Contribute to healthcare professional education about patient advocacy

> *Community Leadership Development: "Based on my advocacy experiences and network development, how can I contribute to community health improvement efforts? What leadership opportunities would effectively use my advocacy expertise to benefit others facing similar healthcare challenges?"*

Measuring Network Effectiveness and Health Outcomes

Network Performance Assessment

Relationship Quality Evaluation

Regularly assess the effectiveness of your health advocacy network:

Information and Support Quality. Evaluate quality of information and support received from network connections.
Goal-Achievement Effectiveness. Measure effectiveness of network relationships in achieving health goals.
Mutual Benefit Levels. Assess mutual benefit levels in professional and peer relationships.
Network Diversity. Review network diversity and comprehensiveness for your health needs.

Health Outcome Correlation

Track how network development correlates with health outcome improvements:

Access and Quality via Network. Track healthcare access and quality improvements through network connections.
Earlier Detection Success. Measure earlier detection or intervention success through network research and resources.
Network-Supported Treatment Gains. Identify treatment effectiveness improvements through network-supported advocacy.
Quality of Life Enhancements. Note quality of life enhancements through peer support and professional partnerships.

Network Assessment Framework: "Help me develop metrics for evaluating the effectiveness of my health advocacy network. What indicators suggest that network relationships are contributing to better health outcomes and more effective advocacy?"

Continuous Network Optimization

Strategic Network Expansion

Identify gaps in your network and opportunities for strategic expansion:

Unrepresented Specialties. Add healthcare specialties or expertise areas not adequately represented in your network.
Diversity Expansion. Pursue geographic or demographic diversity that might provide additional perspectives.
Research and Advocacy Resources. Add research or advocacy resources that could enhance network effectiveness.
Access-Improving Relationships. Build professional relationships that might improve healthcare access or quality.

Network Pruning and Refinement

Regularly evaluate network relationships for ongoing value:

Low-Benefit Relationships. Prune relationships that no longer provide mutual benefit or support.
Unreliable Sources. Remove information sources that have become less reliable or relevant.
Non-Collaborative Connections. Let go of professional connections that don't support collaborative healthcare.
Non-Evidence-Based Communities. Step away from communities that don't maintain evidence-based approaches to health advocacy.

Technology and Future Innovation Integration

Emerging Technology Evaluation

Health Innovation Assessment

Develop frameworks for evaluating new health technologies and approaches:

Evidence Base. Evaluate evidence base and research support for new innovations.
Safety Profiles. Review safety profiles and potential risks of emerging treatments.
Cost and Accessibility. Consider cost-effectiveness and accessibility considerations.
Integration Potential. Assess integration potential with existing health optimization strategies.

AI and Healthcare Evolution

Prepare for continued evolution in AI applications to healthcare:

Personal Health AI. Anticipate personal health AI that provides increasingly sophisticated analysis.
Healthcare Delivery AI. Monitor healthcare delivery AI that may improve or potentially bias care access.
Research AI. Watch research AI that accelerates medical knowledge development.
Advocacy AI. Support advocacy AI that supports patient rights and healthcare navigation.

> *Future Technology Strategy: "Help me develop an approach to evaluating and potentially integrating emerging health technologies*

and AI developments. What criteria should guide decisions about adopting new health innovations, and how can I stay informed about developments most relevant to my health profile?"

Sustainable Advocacy and Network Development

Long-Term Sustainability Planning

Advocacy Skill Maintenance

Develop systems for maintaining and improving advocacy skills over time:

Regular Approach Review. Conduct regular review and updating of advocacy approaches based on outcomes.
Continued Education. Pursue continued education about healthcare systems and innovations.
Skill Sharing. Engage in skill sharing with other advocates for mutual improvement.
Professional Development. Invest in professional development in health advocacy and communication.

Network Sustainability

Create approaches that maintain network value over time:

Regular Contribution. Make regular contributions to network relationships and communities.
Succession Planning. Engage in succession planning for leadership roles in advocacy organizations.

Mentor for Continuity. Mentor new advocates to ensure community continuity.
Document for Future Advocates. Document successful strategies for future advocates.

Legacy and Impact Considerations

Systemic Impact Development

Consider how your advocacy network contributes to broader healthcare improvements:

Share Successful Strategies. Document and share successful advocacy strategies widely.
Contribute to Equity Research. Contribute to research on healthcare equity and patient advocacy.
Policy Advocacy. Engage in policy advocacy that benefits broader communities.
Provider Education. Support professional education that improves healthcare provider patient advocacy.

Knowledge Transfer and Continuity

Ensure that advocacy knowledge and network relationships benefit future advocates:

Systematic Documentation. Maintain systematic documentation of advocacy approaches and outcomes.
Mentoring Programs. Develop mentoring programs for new patient advocates.
Resource Development. Build resource development that supports ongoing community advocacy.

Organizational Integration. Integrate with established advocacy organizations for sustainability.

Legacy Planning Analysis: "Help me consider how my health advocacy network and expertise can contribute to lasting improvements in healthcare equity and patient advocacy. What approaches ensure that my advocacy experience benefits others facing similar challenges long-term?"

From Individual Advocacy to Collective Health Transformation

Building your personal health intelligence network transforms individual advocacy into a powerful force for both personal health optimization and systemic healthcare improvement. The networks you develop provide access to cutting-edge research, supportive peer relationships, collaborative professional partnerships, and opportunities for contributing to healthcare equity for broader communities.

The comprehensive network outlined in this chapter provides multiple pathways for achieving health goals: research access that keeps you informed about innovations, peer support that validates and enhances your advocacy efforts, professional relationships that improve care quality, and community connections that amplify individual advocacy into collective action.

Your health intelligence network becomes a living system that evolves with your health needs, incorporates new research and technologies, and provides ongoing support for navigation of complex healthcare challenges. This network approach ensures that your advocacy efforts remain current, effective, and sustainable over time.

Remember that the most powerful health advocacy networks balance individual benefit with collective contribution. Your experiences navigating healthcare bias, developing advocacy skills, and achieving better health outcomes provide valuable insights that can benefit others facing similar challenges. The network you build serves not only your health optimization but also contributes to broader healthcare transformation.

The journey from passive patient to sophisticated health advocate culminates in this network development stage, where individual advocacy becomes part of a broader movement toward healthcare equity, patient empowerment, and systemic improvement. Your health intelligence network represents both the culmination of your advocacy development and the foundation for ongoing health optimization and community contribution.

Through the comprehensive AI-enhanced healthcare advocacy framework outlined in this book, you now possess the tools, strategies, and networks necessary to achieve optimal health outcomes while contributing to healthcare improvements that benefit entire communities. Your healthcare war room is complete, and your mission to transform healthcare through informed advocacy continues.

Exercise 11.1 – Your 90-Day Health Intelligence Plan

Write down three specific actions you will take in the next 90 days to build your personal health intelligence network. Include dates, specific people to contact, and measurable outcomes.

Reflection: *Which of these actions scares you the most? That's probably the one you need to do first.*

Exercise 11.2 – Your Letter to Future You

Write a letter to yourself to be read in one year. Tell future-you what you hope to have accomplished, what you're committing to change, and what you want to remember about why this work matters.

____

____

____

____

____

____

____

____

____

____

____

____

Reflection: *If you do nothing different after finishing this book, what will your health look like in one year? What if you do everything you've committed to?*

100 AI Health Prompts for Daily Health Intelligence

A Companion Guide to AI Healthcare War Room

Disclaimer: These prompts are for educational and self-advocacy purposes only. They are not intended to replace professional medical advice, diagnosis, or treatment. Always consult with qualified healthcare providers for medical concerns.

How to Use These Prompts

Each prompt is designed to help you gather information, analyze patterns, and prepare for healthcare conversations. Replace bracketed placeholders with your specific information. Use these prompts with AI tools like ChatGPT, Claude, or Perplexity AI for research and analysis.

Section 1: Daily Health Monitoring & Analysis (Prompts 1-20)

Symptom Tracking & Pattern Recognition

1. **Daily Symptom Analysis** "Analyze this symptom pattern from today: [describe symptoms, timing, severity, triggers]. What potential causes should I research, and what patterns might indicate need for medical attention?"

2. **Weekly Symptom Trending** "Compare my symptoms from this week [provide daily summaries] to identify patterns. What trends suggest improvement, worsening, or cyclical patterns that might guide treatment decisions?"

3. **Trigger Identification** "Help me identify potential triggers for these symptoms: [list symptoms]. Based on my activities today [describe food, sleep, stress, environment], what correlations should I investigate?"

4. **Symptom Severity Scaling** "Create a personalized symptom severity scale for [specific condition/symptoms]. Help me describe severity levels that healthcare providers will understand and take seriously."

5. **Sleep Quality Impact Analysis** "Analyze how my sleep pattern [describe duration, quality, timing] might be affecting these health issues: [list current symptoms/conditions]. What sleep optimizations might improve my symptoms?"

6. **Energy Level Correlation** "Track the relationship between my energy levels [describe pattern] and these factors: [diet, exercise, stress, symptoms]. What patterns suggest actionable improvements?"

7. **Mood and Physical Health Connection** "Examine connections between my mood patterns [describe] and physical symptoms [list symptoms]. What relationships might indicate underlying health issues worth investigating?"

8. **Exercise Response Analysis** "Analyze how different types of exercise affect my symptoms: [describe exercise types and symptom responses]. What exercise modifications might optimize my health outcomes?"

9. **Hydration Impact Assessment** "Evaluate how my hydration levels [describe intake patterns] correlate with these symptoms: [list symptoms]. What hydration strategies might improve my overall health?"

10. **Environmental Factor Analysis** "Analyze how environmental factors [weather, air quality, location changes] affect my symptoms: [describe symptom variations]. What environmental modifications might help?"

Nutrition & Dietary Analysis

11. **Daily Nutrition Impact** "Analyze how today's food choices [list foods with timing] might affect my health conditions: [list conditions]. What nutritional adjustments could optimize my health?"

12. **Food Trigger Identification** "Help me identify potential food triggers for these symptoms: [list symptoms]. Based on my recent diet [describe foods], what elimination approach might be helpful?"

13. **Nutrient Deficiency Investigation** "Based on my diet patterns [describe typical foods] and symptoms [list symptoms], what nutrient deficiencies should I investigate with my healthcare provider?"

14. **Meal Timing Optimization** "Analyze how my meal timing [describe eating schedule] affects my energy, symptoms, and sleep. What timing adjustments might improve my health outcomes?"

15. Blood Sugar Impact Assessment "Evaluate how my food choices today [list foods with timing] might affect blood sugar stability, given my symptoms: [describe energy crashes, mood changes, etc.]."

Medication & Supplement Tracking

16. Medication Response Monitoring "Track my response to [medication name and dosage] over [time period]. Based on these symptoms/improvements [describe], what should I discuss with my prescriber?"

17. Supplement Effectiveness Analysis "Analyze the effectiveness of my current supplements [list supplements with dosages] for my health goals [describe goals]. What changes might optimize outcomes?"

18. Side Effect Pattern Recognition "Help me determine if these symptoms [describe symptoms] might be related to my medications [list medications] or indicate other health issues requiring investigation."

19. Drug Interaction Research "Research potential interactions between my medications [list] and supplements [list]. What combinations require medical monitoring or adjustment?"

20. Timing Optimization for Medications "Optimize the timing of my medications and supplements [list with current timing] to maximize effectiveness and minimize side effects."

Section 2: Healthcare Preparation & Advocacy (Prompts 21-40)

Appointment Preparation

21. **Pre-Appointment Research** "Prepare me for my appointment about [condition/symptoms]. What questions should I ask, what information should I bring, and what outcomes should I advocate for?"

22. **Symptom Summary Creation** "Create a professional medical summary of my symptoms: [describe symptoms with timeline]. Organize this for clear communication with my healthcare provider."

23. **Family History Medical Relevance** "Analyze my family health history [provide relevant details] for connections to my current symptoms [describe]. What patterns should I highlight to my doctor?"

24. **Test Result Preparation Questions** "I'm receiving lab results for [tests performed]. Based on my symptoms [describe] and demographics [age/gender], what questions should I ask about the results?"

25. **Second Opinion Preparation** "Prepare me to seek a second opinion about [diagnosis/treatment recommendation]. What information should I gather, and how should I present my case?"

Medical Communication

26. **Provider Communication Strategy** "Help me communicate these concerns [describe] to my healthcare provider in a way that encourages thorough evaluation rather than dismissal."

27. Medical Terminology Research "Research appropriate medical terminology for describing these symptoms: [describe in lay terms]. Help me communicate more effectively with healthcare providers."

28. Treatment Option Discussion Prep "Prepare me to discuss treatment options for [condition] with my doctor. What questions ensure I understand all available approaches and their trade-offs?"

29. Specialist Referral Advocacy "Help me advocate for a referral to [specialist type] for my symptoms: [describe]. What medical justification supports this referral request?"

30. Insurance Authorization Support "Draft a letter supporting medical necessity for [treatment/test] for my condition [describe condition and symptoms]. Include relevant medical guidelines and research."

Bias Recognition & Response

31. Gaslighting Response Preparation "Prepare responses to potential medical gaslighting phrases like '[specific dismissive statement]' regarding my symptoms: [describe symptoms]."

32. Bias Pattern Documentation "Analyze this healthcare interaction [describe interaction] for potential bias. What patterns suggest inappropriate dismissal of my concerns?"

33. Evidence-Based Advocacy "Create evidence-based arguments for why my symptoms [describe] warrant investigation, particularly given potential bias against [my demographic characteristics]."

34. Alternative Provider Research "Research healthcare providers in [location/specialty] who demonstrate awareness of healthcare bias and practice patient-centered care for people with my profile."

35. Systematic Documentation Strategy "Create a documentation system for tracking healthcare interactions that ensures I can identify patterns of bias and advocate effectively for appropriate care."

Research & Validation

36. Symptom Validation Research "Research medical literature validating these symptoms: [describe symptoms] as legitimate medical concerns requiring investigation, particularly in [my demographic]."

37. Demographic-Specific Research "Find research on how [condition/symptoms] present in [my demographic characteristics]. What studies show different presentation patterns I should discuss with providers?"

38. Treatment Effectiveness Research "Research treatment effectiveness for [condition] in people with my characteristics: [relevant demographics]. What approaches show strongest evidence for people like me?"

39. Alternative Diagnostic Approaches "Research alternative diagnostic approaches for [symptoms/suspected condition] that might be more appropriate than standard protocols for someone with my profile."

40. Healthcare Disparity Research "Research healthcare disparities affecting [my demographic] for [type of condition]. What studies document bias that might affect my care?"

Section 3: Family Health Intelligence (Prompts 41-60)

Family Pattern Analysis

41. **Genetic vs Environmental Analysis** "Analyze this family health pattern [describe conditions affecting multiple relatives] to distinguish between genetic predisposition and environmental factors."

42. **Generational Health Trends** "Compare health patterns across generations in my family [provide details]. What trends suggest environmental changes or improved/worsened health trajectories?"

43. **Gender-Specific Family Patterns** "Analyze health conditions affecting women vs men in my family [provide details]. What gender-specific risks should guide my prevention strategies?"

44. **Timing Pattern Recognition** "Identify timing patterns in my family health history [provide ages of onset for various conditions]. What patterns suggest optimal screening or prevention timing for me?"

45. **Environmental Exposure Analysis** "Research potential environmental health factors affecting my family based on geographic locations [list places] and occupational exposures [list occupations] across generations."

Risk Assessment & Prevention

46. **Personal Risk Stratification** "Based on my family history [provide details] and current health status [describe], stratify my risk levels for various conditions and recommend prevention strategies."

47. Screening Schedule Optimization "Create an optimal screening schedule for me based on family health patterns [provide details] and current medical guidelines for someone with my risk profile."

48. Lifestyle Prevention Planning "Develop lifestyle prevention strategies based on my family health patterns [describe] and current research on preventing these conditions in people with my background."

49. Early Detection Strategy "Based on family patterns of [specific conditions], what early detection strategies and warning signs should I monitor throughout different life stages?"

50. Protective Factor Analysis "Analyze what factors may have protected certain family members from developing conditions that affected others. How can I apply these protective strategies?"

Medical Communication

51. Family History Medical Summary "Create a professional family health history summary for my healthcare providers that highlights clinically relevant patterns and risks requiring attention."

52. Genetic Counseling Preparation "Prepare me for genetic counseling based on my family history [provide details]. What questions should I ask and what outcomes should I seek?"

53. Specialist Consultation Strategy "Based on family health patterns [describe], which specialists should I consult preventively, and how should I present my family history to them?"

54. Insurance Coverage Advocacy "Help me advocate for insurance coverage of preventive testing based on my family history [provide details]. What documentation supports medical necessity?"

55. Risk Communication with Family "Help me communicate health risks and prevention strategies to family members based on our shared family health patterns [describe patterns]."

Research Integration

56. Hereditary Research Updates "Research current understanding of hereditary factors for conditions in my family [list conditions]. What new research might change prevention or treatment approaches?"

57. Epigenetic Factor Research "Research how environmental factors might influence genetic expression for conditions in my family history [list conditions]. What lifestyle factors might modify genetic risk?"

58. Precision Medicine Opportunities "Research precision medicine approaches relevant to my family health profile [describe]. What genetic testing or personalized treatments might be beneficial?"

59. Family Health Database Management "Create a systematic approach to maintaining and updating family health information. What data should I collect and how should I organize it for medical use?"

60. Multigenerational Health Planning "Develop a multigenerational health strategy that considers family patterns [describe] and prepares for health needs across different life stages."

Section 4: Lab Results & Health Data Analysis (Prompts 61-80)

Lab Result Interpretation

61. **Comprehensive Lab Analysis** "Analyze these lab results [provide specific values] for optimal ranges rather than just normal ranges, considering my age, gender, and health goals."

62. **Trending Pattern Recognition** "Compare these lab values over time [provide historical data] to identify concerning trends, improvements, or patterns requiring attention."

63. **Demographic-Specific Optimization** "Research optimal lab value ranges for [specific tests] in someone with my demographics [age/gender/ethnicity]. How do these compare to my current results?"

64. **Correlation Analysis** "Analyze relationships between these different lab values [provide multiple results]. What patterns might indicate metabolic dysfunction or emerging health issues?"

65. **Symptom-Lab Correlation** "Correlate my lab results [provide values] with my current symptoms [describe symptoms]. What connections might explain my symptom pattern?"

Early Detection Analysis

66. **Subclinical Dysfunction Recognition** "Based on these lab trends [provide data], what subclinical health issues might be developing before they become symptomatic?"

67. **Metabolic Health Assessment** "Analyze these metabolic markers [provide relevant lab values] for early signs of insulin resistance, inflammation, or cardiovascular risk."

68. **Nutritional Status Evaluation** "Evaluate my nutritional status based on these lab values [provide relevant results]. What deficiencies or imbalances might require intervention?"

69. **Thyroid Function Optimization** "Analyze my thyroid function tests [provide values] for optimal function rather than just normal function. What patterns suggest need for optimization?"

70. **Inflammatory Marker Assessment** "Interpret these inflammatory markers [provide values] in the context of my symptoms [describe] and family history [relevant details]."

Intervention Planning

71. **Lab-Guided Supplement Strategy** "Based on these lab results [provide values] and my health goals [describe], what supplement interventions might optimize my health markers?"

72. **Dietary Modification Strategy** "Using these lab results [provide relevant values], what dietary modifications might improve my health markers and address any deficiencies or imbalances?"

73. **Exercise Prescription Optimization** "Based on my lab values [provide relevant results] and current fitness level [describe], what exercise approaches might optimize my health markers?"

74. **Monitoring Schedule Planning** "Based on these lab trends [provide data] and my risk factors [describe], what monitoring schedule would help track improvements and catch problems early?"

75. Provider Discussion Preparation "Prepare me to discuss these lab results [provide values] with my healthcare provider, focusing on optimization opportunities and concerning trends."

Advanced Analysis

76. Functional Medicine Interpretation "Analyze these lab results [provide values] from a functional medicine perspective, focusing on optimal function rather than just disease absence."

77. Biomarker Integration Analysis "Integrate these various biomarkers [provide different test results] to create a comprehensive picture of my health status and optimization opportunities."

78. Risk Stratification Assessment "Use these lab values [provide results] to assess my risk levels for various conditions and recommend targeted prevention strategies."

79. Personalized Medicine Applications "Research how these lab results [provide values] and my genetic background [if known] might guide personalized treatment or prevention approaches."

80. Quality of Life Correlation "Correlate these objective lab measures [provide values] with my subjective quality of life indicators [describe symptoms, energy, mood] to identify optimization targets."

Section 5: Lifestyle Optimization & Integration (Prompts 81-100)

Holistic Lifestyle Analysis

81. **Comprehensive Lifestyle Assessment** "Analyze how my current lifestyle patterns [describe diet, exercise, sleep, stress management] might be affecting my health conditions [list conditions]."

82. **Stress-Health Connection Analysis** "Evaluate how my stress patterns [describe stress sources and responses] correlate with my health symptoms [describe] and identify stress management strategies."

83. **Sleep Optimization Strategy** "Based on my sleep patterns [describe current sleep habits] and health goals [describe], create a comprehensive sleep optimization plan."

84. **Environmental Health Assessment** "Assess how my living and working environments [describe] might affect my health conditions [list] and recommend environmental modifications."

85. **Social Health Integration** "Analyze how my social connections and support systems [describe] affect my health outcomes and recommend strategies for social health optimization."

Personalized Intervention Planning

86. **Individualized Exercise Prescription** "Create an exercise plan tailored to my health conditions [list], fitness level [describe], and health goals [describe], considering any limitations or modifications needed."

87. **Personalized Nutrition Strategy** "Develop a nutrition plan based on my health conditions [list], food preferences [describe], and optimization goals [describe], considering any dietary restrictions."

88. **Stress Management Customization** "Create personalized stress management strategies based on my stress triggers [describe], personality type [describe], and lifestyle constraints [describe]."

89. **Recovery and Restoration Planning** "Design recovery strategies appropriate for my health conditions [list] and lifestyle demands [describe] to optimize healing and prevent burnout."

90. **Habit Formation Strategy** "Create a systematic approach to implementing healthy lifestyle changes [describe desired changes] considering my current habits [describe] and potential barriers [describe]."

Long-term Optimization

91. **Life Stage Health Planning** "Develop health optimization strategies appropriate for my current life stage [describe age and circumstances] and prepare for future health needs."

92. **Seasonal Health Adaptation** "Create strategies for adapting my health routines [describe current routines] to seasonal changes and their effects on my health conditions [describe]."

93. **Travel Health Maintenance** "Develop strategies for maintaining my health routines [describe] and managing my health conditions [list] while traveling or during schedule disruptions."

94. **Technology Integration for Health** "Recommend health technology tools and apps that would support my health goals [describe] and integrate well with my lifestyle [describe]."

95. Health Goal Prioritization "Help me prioritize my health goals [list multiple goals] based on my current health status [describe] and create a realistic implementation timeline."

Integration & Sustainability

96. Holistic Health Integration "Create a comprehensive health plan that integrates medical care [describe current care], lifestyle modifications [describe], and self-advocacy strategies."

97. Support System Development "Identify types of support [medical, social, professional] I need to sustain my health optimization efforts and achieve my health goals [describe]."

98. Progress Monitoring System "Design a system for tracking progress toward my health goals [describe goals] that includes both objective measures and subjective quality of life indicators."

99. Obstacle Anticipation Planning "Identify potential obstacles to my health optimization efforts [consider lifestyle, medical, social factors] and develop contingency strategies."

100. Legacy Health Planning "Create a long-term health strategy that considers my family health patterns [describe], personal health goals [describe], and desired health legacy for future generations."

Tips for Effective Prompt Usage

Prompt Customization

Replace Placeholders. Replace all bracketed placeholders with your specific information before using any prompt.
Modify for Your Situation. Modify prompts to match your particular health concerns and goals.
Combine Prompts. Combine prompts when addressing complex health situations that require multiple angles.

Research Integration

Cross-Reference AI Tools. Use multiple AI tools to cross-reference information for greater reliability.
Verify with Medical Sources. Always verify AI-generated health information with reputable medical sources.
Use for Preparation, Not Diagnosis. Focus on using prompts to organize your thoughts and prepare questions rather than for medical diagnosis.

Documentation and Tracking

Record Insights. Keep records of insights gained from using these prompts.
Track Useful Prompts. Track which prompts provide the most useful information for your situation.
Share with Providers. Share relevant insights with your healthcare providers during appointments.

Download the Rhythm by Womb WatchAI® App. Download the Rhythm by Womb WatchAI® App to put these prompts to work in your daily health routine.

Safety Considerations

Not a Substitute for Medical Advice. Never use AI responses as a substitute for professional medical advice.

Seek Emergency Care When Needed. Seek immediate medical attention for emergency symptoms.

Consult Qualified Providers. Always consult with qualified healthcare providers before making significant health decisions.

Remember: These prompts are tools for self-advocacy and health optimization, not for medical diagnosis or treatment. Your healthcare journey requires collaboration with qualified medical professionals who can provide personalized medical advice based on your complete health picture.

About the Author

QUANDA FRANCIS, MBA is a serial entrepreneur, multi-patent inventor, and the founder of Womb WatchAI Corp., a biotechnology company focused on women's health.

Her journey began the way too many women's stories do — with a healthcare system that nearly killed her. After almost dying during childbirth and enduring years of continuous misdiagnosis, Quanda made a decision that would change the trajectory of women's healthcare technology: she would build the tools she wished had existed when she needed them most. That decision became Womb WatchAI Corp.

Today, Quanda is the architect of an entire ecosystem of AI-powered women's health technology, including Rhythm by Womb WatchAI®, the app launching May 2026 that allows women to apply the tactical strategies in this book to monitor and advocate for their own health in real time. Rhythm represents the practical extension of everything you have just read — the moment where the playbook becomes a daily practice.

As a multi-patent inventor, Quanda holds intellectual property in bio-intent orchestration systems, dynamic AI agent creation for women's health, and adaptive sensor fusion technology. Her work sits at the intersection of artificial intelligence, biotechnology, and the lived reality of women who have been told their pain is imaginary, their symptoms are exaggerated, and their concerns are not worth investigating.

Quanda has built a global audience of women who refuse to accept dismissal as a diagnosis. Through her viral healthcare advocacy, she has reached millions with evidence-based strategies for navigating medical bias, decoding lab results, and using AI as a strategic ally in healthcare conversations. Her message is simple and uncompromising: women deserve healthcare that was designed with their bodies in mind, and until the system delivers it, women will build the tools to deliver it themselves.

She holds an MBA and brings the discipline of strategic business thinking to a field that has historically been dominated by clinical perspectives that overlooked women entirely. Her work has been recognized by NVIDIA Inception and Google for Startups, and Womb WatchAI Corp. is positioned to become a category-defining platform in women's health technology.

When she is not building companies, filing patents, or writing books, Quanda is doing what she does best: refusing to be told what is impossible. This book is proof that one woman with a laptop, a story, and a refusal to be ignored can change how healthcare works for millions.

She wrote this book for her grandmother, Janie. She wrote it for every woman who has been dismissed. And she wrote it for every woman who is about to walk into a doctor's appointment and needs a tactical plan to be heard.

Connect with Quanda Francis & WOMB WATCHAI®

Continue Your War Room

Get the AI Healthcare War Room Companion Journal — 90 days of guided tracking that builds on every exercise in this book, so you walk into every appointment armed with three months of receipts your doctor cannot dismiss.

Available in hardcover at www.rhythmbywombwatchai.com/journal

Download Rhythm by WOMB WATCHAI®

The AI health advisor that decodes your lab results, tracks your cycle, analyzes your symptoms, and turns every signal your body sends into the answers you've been waiting your entire life to hear.

Free for 7 days. Available on the App Store and Google Play.
www.rhythmbywombwatchai.com

Stay Connected

Personal Website: www.quandafrancis.com

LIV by WOMB WATCHAI® — the community blog featuring stories, research, and conversations on women's health: www.wombwatchai.app/liv-by-wombwatchai

WOMB WATCHAI® corporate home: www.wombwatchai.com

www.ingramcontent.com/pod-product-compliance
Lightning Source LLC
LaVergne TN
LVHW090105250926
848814LV00044B/12